ALL
ABOUT
BLUE
CRABS

AND HOW TO CATCH THEM

BY RUSSELL ROBERTS

Published by Centennial Publications
Copyright © 1993 Russell Roberts
ISBN #1-882418-07-7

DEDICATION

This book is dedicated to my grandfather, who introduced a young boy to the wonders of the sea and to the excitement and mystery of the greatest sport in the world, crabbing. I would give all that I possess to turn back time and spend just one more golden day with him on the sun drenched waters of the Manasquan River.

CONTENTS

Artwork by Connie Moller
Photos by Pat King–Roberts

Introduction

The Remarkable Blue Crab

Consider, for a moment, the remarkable blue crab. First of all, consider how remarkable it is that there are any blue crabs to catch at all. Out of hundreds of thousands, even millions, of eggs laid by a single female, just a minuscule fraction survive to become adults.

After being born, the "baby" crabs must pass through numerous growth stages before reaching adulthood. Their theme song during this time could easily be *Growing Up Is Hard To Do,* because while they struggle to grow they are extremely vulnerable to a score of water-dwelling predators, as well as to random environmental factors such as water salinity and temperature.

If the young blue crab is lucky enough to survive all these obstacles, it is still not home free. In order to continue growing the crab must shed its shell many times by a process known as moulting. Each moult leaves the crab weak and helpless for several hours – easy prey not only for predators but also for man, who pursues softshell crabs with a Holy Grail–like fervor.

Only if it survives all of this, and the odds are nothing you would want to take to Las Vegas, does the blue crab become the thick-clawed, hard-shelled, feisty beauty that is such a thrill to catch – and eat. Remarkable.

Next consider how remarkable it is that you can even make such a catch at all. Although a blue crab will never beat a dolphin in an intelligence test, the crab is a clever, elusive adversary. Skittish as a colt and quick as lightning, the blue crab's unpredictability gives even the most veteran crabbers apoplexy.

For you and I, the recreational crabbers, it is even worse. Unlike fishermen, we do not have the luxury of efficient hooks or gaudy, scientifically-tested lures to attract the prey and hold it fast once it takes the bait. Instead, we must hope that the crab is sufficiently interested in the bait to not only take it, but to remain with it. And since the bait is usually just an ordinary piece of fish or chicken, it must compete with everything else on the bottom – other crabs, sea grass, live fish, dead fish, rocks, debris and so on – for the crab's attention. Even once you have managed to attract the crab, and it is happily tearing at your bait, there are more pitfalls to overcome before the blue crab winds up in your bushel basket. As you try to bring the crab in, one small slip-up – an inadvertent jerk of a dropline, a hole in a scoop net, a malfunctioning trap, the waves of a passing boat stirring the water, a sudden flash of sunlight – will send the crab rocketing away, leaving you with nothing but a chewed–up piece of bait for your trouble. Yet recreational crabbers haul in countless bushel baskets of blue crabs every year. Remarkable.

Finally, think of the amazing blue crab itself. Although dwarfed in size by many other aquatic creatures, the blue crab backs down from no one, be it natural predator or man. It is truly one of nature's most irascible creatures, ready to fight no matter how steep the odds or how formidable the foe. The crab's claws flash out at incredible speed, and woe to the fish or finger that gets caught in their vise-like grip.

As if this impressive weapon was not enough, the blue crab is one of the speediest swimmers in the water, and can disappear faster than your money at income tax time. It is not exactly helpless on land either, as anyone who has ever pursued a crab scuttling madly across the sand can attest.

Even the fact that the blue crab is still with us is surprising. While other creatures have decreased in population over the years, either through over-harvesting or the changing environment, the blue crab has not only survived, but prospered. The crab population has remained steady, despite the increased demand for crab meat. As for the crab itself, it is still the same quick, resourceful, ill-tempered and tasty creature that it was hundreds of years ago.

In fact, if it wasn't for the blue crab's melt-in-your–mouth taste, it is very probable that man would have long ago decided to leave this cantankerous creature alone. But there's good reason that part of this crab's scientific name means "tasty." The blue crab is prized so highly as food that it practically supports one entire region of the country and contributes greatly to the enjoyment and pleasure of people from Massachusetts to Texas. All of this because of the tiny but mighty blue crab. And that, quite simply, is remarkable.

This book is about that amazing crab – not only about how to catch it, but also about how it lives and what it likes, and doesn't like.

Because crabs and crabbing should be fun, there's some information on how people have regarded crabs throughout the centuries, and a glossary of "crab talk" so you can speak to either a marine scientist or a crusty old bayman on equal terms. Since it doesn't make much sense to catch crabs unless you're going to eat them, the book also contains tips on how to prepare and cook crabs, as well as a few basic recipes to get you started in the kitchen. Finally, because crabbing is truly something that can be shared with your children and your children's children, there is a story about how a wise old man once handed down his particular crabbing skills to a wide-eyed boy.

Crabbing should be fun. It's not a hard sport to get started in, nor a hard sport to learn. Too many times people make crabbing out to be some big mystery, and throw a lot of jargon and data around to prove their point. The purpose of this book is to build your confidence so that you'll go out and try crabbing. After that, you'll learn quickly enough where and how to catch blue crabs without worring about a host of other factors, and without losing the fun and the magic of crabbing.

There *is* magic in crabbing, particularly if you're experiencing for the first time the defiant tug of resistance when the crab hits the bait on your dropline and you know that you've "got one."

It is the magic of a summer day spent on the water, with a lazy breeze tousling your hair and the tangy smell of salt air invigorating your senses. It is the magic of feeling, deep inside, that maybe, just maybe, this is what life was meant to be all about.

And that's more than remarkable. That's wonderful.

Chapter One
The Beautiful, Savory Swimmer

The world is full of crabs. No, that's not a personal comment about people, but rather an observation on the incredible number and variety of crabs that exist. There are hundreds of different types of crabs roaming about the earth, in all shapes, colors and sizes. Some, like hermit crabs, are so small and familiar to us that we think nothing about picking them up or keeping them as pets. But others, like the mighty king crab with its long, spider-like legs, are much less "cuddly."

It might seem impossible that the cute little hermit crab is the cousin of the ill-tempered blue crab, but it illustrates how different the crab species is. Maybe nowhere else in the animal kingdom can you find such a broad diversity of attitudes and appearances as in the crab family.

Need a different color crab? Try the reddish pebble crab, the lavender iridescent swimming crab, the aptly-named green crab, the sky-colored claws of the blue crab, or the pale yellow ghost crab. Coral crabs, which live in tropical waters, come in a dazzling variety of rainbow colors, including orange, blue, white and red.

Crabs are just as varied when it comes to shape and size. You probably know what a blue crab looks like, but isn't it hard to believe it bears any relation to the hideously ugly spider crab, with its gangly legs and pear-shaped body? And what about the delicate arrow crab? It's almost impossible to believe that this graceful creature is related to the lumbering, squat stone crab.

As far as movement goes, the crab family seems to again have all bases covered. Our typical perception of how crabs move is the frantic sideways scuttling motion common to the blue crab, among others. But a ghost crab tiptoes across the sand as if walking on eggshells, its movements strongly suggestive of old cartoons that show a man sneaking into the house late at night with his shoes in hand, trying not to awaken his sleeping wife. Since there are so many different types of crabs, it seems only right that crabs can be found practically everywhere: beaches, sand dunes, rocks, and the water are all habitats for various crab species. Crabs also have a bewildering variety of ways to escape from their enemies, besides the tried and true method of fighting with their claws. Some crabs burrow into the mud so that only their eyes are poking up above ground. Sponge crabs cut off a piece of sponge and carry it around on their backs so that they blend perfectly into the background. Other crab species go this one better by carrying sea anemones (small creatures with poison in their tentacles) on their back, so that attackers not only get pinched but stung as well. A species of crab in the Indian Ocean has a body that is sculptured like a piece of coral that inhabits the reefs where it lives – the perfect camouflage.

But sometimes, despite all their precautions, crabs do get caught by predators. If the crab has been seized by an appendage (leg, claw, swimming fin, etc.), it has one last-ditch defense: it can break off the captured limb and dart away. Crabs can pull this Houdini–like escape because their appendages come equipped with what are called *breaking planes:* areas that are designed to break off without injuring the crab. A crab can break off its limbs merely by tightening its muscles in a particular fashion. The limb falls off and a blood clot almost immediately seals off the wound. Later, a new limb will start to grow in the missing one's place. This process is called regeneration.

Colorful, different in size and shape, possessing the ability to grow new limbs in place of old – crabs are indeed amazing creatures. And, just when you think you've seen it all, watch a coconut crab climb a tree to pick a ripe coconut for its dinner and then back down the same tree without ever dropping the coconut. It'll make you think crabs can do anything!

But despite all the diverse and unique crabs in the world, this book is concerned with just one: the blue crab.

Rarely has an animal species been so celebrated as the blue crab. It virtually supports the economy of one entire region of the United States – the Chesapeake Bay area (a staggering ninety percent of the total crab catch in America comes from the

Chesapeake) – and it gives immense pleasure to people up and down the Atlantic seaboard and all the way along the Gulf Coast. But why stop there? Although initially confined to the Western Atlantic Ocean, the blue crab has now spread all over the world. You can drop a baited line in the waters of the Red Sea, on the Pacific coast of the United States, and even in the Indian Ocean, and you'd have a better than average chance of catching a blue crab. It's fast becoming an international star. And because it's so well known, almost everyone recognizes a blue crab when they see it. Blue crabs have ten appendages – five on each side of their body. It is from these that they get much of their amazing ability. The first appendage is the one we're most familiar with: the claw. The top part of the claw closes on the bottom, and if you've ever been unfortunate enough to have your finger or toe between the two when they come together, you know the power that even a tiny crab has. The next three appendages are called walking legs; they help the crab move around, both on land and in water. The last is the swimming paddle; their flat, oar-like tip is what gives the blue crab its jet propulsion through the water. If you've never seen a crab shoot away from you just when you were about to net it, you're going to be surprised at the incredible speed this compact creature possesses.

When scientists want to dine on blue crab they probably order it by its proper name of *Callinectes sapidus*. The first word is Greek for beautiful swimmer, while *sapidus* is Latin for tasty or savory. This is why you'll see the blue crab often referred to as "beautiful savory swimmer," or some such variation. Seldom has a creature been named so accurately. To see a blue crab knifing though the water, with its striking olive-colored shell and its deep blue claws, is truly to see one of Nature's finest creations. Of course, as far as tasty goes, even a single bite of blue crab meat is one of life's great gastronomic pleasures.

What makes blue crabs even more appealing is the fun and challenge of catching them. Crabbing has been called "a poor man's sport" (not wishing to be sexist, we'll alter that a bit to "a poor person's sport"), and it's easy to see why. All you need is some thick twine or string, a long-handled scoop net, and a piece of bait, such as a $2.00 pack of chicken backs and necks from the supermarket, and you're in business. It doesn't take hours of preparation and a bus load of special equipment to catch a crab. As the writer H. L. Mencken once said about crabbing: "Any poor man could go down to the banks of the river, armed with no more than a length of stout cord, a home-made net on a pole, and a chunk of cat's meat, and come home in a couple of hours with enough crabs to feed his family."

The ease and economy of crabbing makes it a sport that cuts across age and social barriers. The person ferreting out blue claws in the lagoon next to you could be a lawyer with a fancy car, or a fry cook at the local fast food restaurant. It doesn't take much for anyone to grab some string, a net and some bait, and head down to the water for a few hours of invigorating fun in the fresh air and sunshine.

Blue crabs help make crabbing fun by being so darn accommodating. You don't have to go to the middle of Chesapeake Bay on the day of the summer equinox and sacrifice a water chestnut in order to find crabs. They're literally everywhere. You can crab from bridges, piers, docks, beaches, boats – you name it, the blue crab's probably there.

Crabs also contribute to the fun of crabbing by having voracious appetites. If crabs were people they'd undoubtedly be teenagers, because their minds are constantly on food. If a crab isn't eating, it's searching for food; and if it isn't doing either, then it's thinking about eating or searching for food.

This, of course, is where you and I come in. By offering the beautiful savory swimmer something to eat, we hope that *we'll* eventually be eating *it*. But before we get down to the particulars of how to catch a blue crab, let's take a fun look at how people over the centuries have viewed this most fascinating of creatures.

Chapter Two

People and Crabs Throughout Time

It might surprise you to learn that, for such a disagreeable and strange looking creature, the crab has been the object of a lot of attention by people and their culture throughout the centuries. Indeed, it might well be the crab's rather odd appearance that has caused it to be of so much interest to so many people in the ancient world. Most other animals that early man came across tended to look essentially the same: a head, two eyes, a mouth, nose, and body, all in basically the same configuration. But the crab was different – much different. It didn't look like anything else walking, running, or even scuttling along. It didn't have a nose or ears, and its mouth was somewhere in the middle of its body. Whether it had teeth or not was anyone's guess, and its eyes – well! Two circular things stuck on the top of stalks and waving around like leaves in a stiff breeze certainly didn't look like the eyes of any other animal.

Most disconcerting of all about the crab's appearance was that it didn't appear to have a head. The eyes and mouth seemed to be coming right out of its body, just like its legs and claws. It looked as strange as a person would with his head coming out of his stomach. Trying to explain about the crab's head, or rather the lack thereof, has given rise to some fascinating and delightful stories, such as the following African folk tale:

In the beginning of time, after making the earth, sky and animals, including the elephant, turtle, leopard and crocodile, Nzambi Mpungu (pronounced n'ZAHM-bee m'POON-goo) began working on yet another creature that she decided to call a crab. But as it was the end of the day, she was tired; she stopped after making the shell and the legs. Before Nzambi Mpungu went to sleep she told the crab to come back in the morning so she could make him a head to go with his fine new body.

All night long the crab boasted to the other animals about how

Nzambi Mpungu was taking two days to make him, instead of one like all the others, and how his head was to be so much more wonderful than any other creature's. By morning a huge crowd of animals had gathered outside Nzambi Mpungu's home to see the glorious head that she was going to give the crab. When she came out of her home the crab pushed his way through the other animals and demanded his splendid new head. But Nzambi Mpungu, angered at how vain and self-important the crab had become, refused to make him a new head. So now, not only is the crab without a head, but he also walks sideways from embarrassment over how all his bragging turned out.

The Chinese attempted to come to grips with the crab's "missing" head through a poem entitled *Old Chang The Crab*:

Old man Chang, I've oft heard it said,
You wear a basket upon your head;
You've two pairs of scissors to cut your meat,
And two pairs of chopsticks with which to eat.

In Japan there are several versions of an ancient fable in which a monkey and a crab become enemies. This happens because the crab asks the monkey to pick some persimmons for it from a tree, but the monkey instead eats the ripe fruit and throws the unripe ones at the crab. One story has the crab holding the monkey in its pinchers until the animal gives it some of its hairs. In other versions the monkey is attacked and ultimately killed by the crab.

Ancient peoples showed how important they felt the crab to be by naming one of the constellations in the sky after a crab (Cancer - Latin for crab), despite the many animals that the early star-gazers could have chosen instead. How Cancer came to be in the sky is explained in Greek mythology: When Hercules was fighting the many-headed Hydra as part of his famous Twelve Labors, a giant crab attempted to aid the Hydra by biting the legendary strongman on the foot. Hercules, however, crushed the crab with one blow of his club, and then killed the Hydra. However, the goddess Hera, ruler of the heavens, lifted the crab into the sky as a reward for its efforts (Hera obviously being unhappy with Hercules at that moment).

Cancer is one of the signs of the zodiac, and people who fall under it are said to like staying home, just like a crab never leaves its shell. Since a crab is soft underneath its hard shell, those born under the sign of Cancer are supposed to be very emotional. Archeological excavations in the Euphrates Valley have uncovered jewelry and coins bearing the likeness of crabs. Crabs appear in paintings and art work from the ancient world. Probably because a crab can grow back lost limbs, Egyptians represented it by the sign of the scarab, which signified immortality. The crab has also been a featured character in literature throughout the ages. One of its most notable appearances was in Rudyard Kipling's famous collection of *Just So Stories*. In "The Crab that Played with the Sea," a large crab gets mad at the Eldest Magician, who during the very beginning of the world makes all the animals beholden to man. The crab goes off and takes refuge in the ocean, where it causes floods and other havoc throughout the world by its constant movement in and out of the water.

When the Eldest Magician finally tracks down the crab and asks it to stop disrupting the earth, the creature is haughty and defiant until the magic man waves a finger and causes the crab's thick shell to drop off, leaving it soft and defenseless. The crab then agrees to leave the sea alone, and receives several gifts, including the ability to hide on land or in water, the use of scissors (claws) to eat and defend itself with, and the return of its hard shell. However, to keep the crab humble, the Eldest Magician decrees that its shell should grow soft every twelve months.

As far as movies go, crabs have a distinction few other animal species have: they were the stars, or rather the bad guys, of the 1950's science fiction film *Attack of the Crab Monsters*. In this movie, crabs on some remote Pacific island were bombarded by that old Cold War bugaboo, atomic radiation. This turned them into giant creatures, who had the distinctly unpleasant habit of eating the heads of humans and then taking on their victim's personalities, including being able to speak telepathically in the recently-digested person's voice. Although the plot is banal and the giant crabs look like walking cardboard, the film is scary in a '50's sort of way.

In order to catch the blue crab, we first have to learn a little bit about its life cycle.

Chapter Three
Mating, Moulting and Maturity

Blue crabs have one of the most interesting life cycles of any creature on this planet. Researchers are only now beginning to understand all the careful and deliberate steps that male and female blue crabs go through before they eventually mate to produce the next generation of hungry crabs that hopefully will be nibbling at your bait in years to come. In fact, before and after mating, male blue crabs are surprisingly considerate of their mates – a trait not normally associated with the cranky and cantankerous crab.

Nature has arranged it so that the sex of blue crabs is about as easy to determine as the weather outside. Just flip a crab over and you can tell by the shape of its apron (abdomen) whether you've caught a *Jimmy* (a male crab) or the opposite sex. The apron of a male crab is long and thin, with a rounded bottom; my grandfather used to call this shape a "candlestick," and it's a fitting description. The apron of an immature female (one that cannot mate) is small and triangular; an immature female is called a *Sally*. However, after the last moult of her life, the female reaches sexual maturity, and the Sally becomes a *sook*. Maturity also brings another change to a female crab besides her name: her apron becomes almost circular.

Besides the apron, there are other significant differences between male and female crabs. Males generally grow larger than females, and have bigger claws as well, although crab size is determined more by the amount of salinity in the water than by sex. Crabs in lower salinity water absorb more water as they go through life, and thus grow larger. That's why where you go crabbing is just as important as how you go crabbing. A big male crab measures between six and eight inches tip to tip; if you catch a female over six, you've got a genuine Big Mama on your hands.

Just as an aside, the largest blue crab ever measured by a

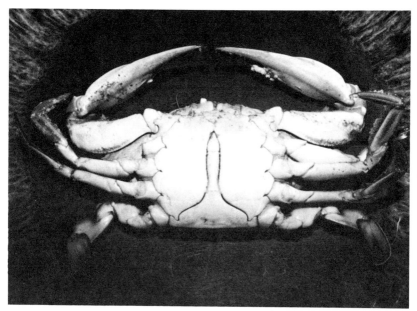

The telltale "candlestick" shape on the apron of a male crab.

The mature female crab has a more rounded apron.

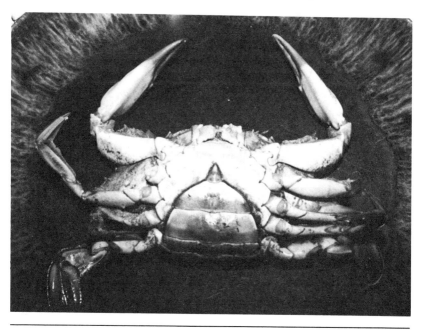

scientist, which means one other than the one your Uncle Charley bagged in the summer of '53, measured 9½ inches in width, and weighed 1½ pounds. From claw tip to claw tip, this behemoth measured 27¾ inches.

Males are also supposed to be smarter and more aggressive than females, according to many old time crabbers, who are also invariably men, so draw your own conclusions here. Another distinction between the two sexes is that the tips of a female's claws are orange/red, while a male's are always blue/purple in color. Veteran crabbers refer to this as a female *painting her nails*. The big lesson from this "battle of the sexes" is that females have less meat in them to eat, not just because they're smaller, but also because their reproductive system takes up more room in their bodies.

What is truly amazing about blue crab reproduction is that they can only mate when a female is moulting, and this act must take place during the female's final moult of her life. Given all these variables, you might wonder how crabs have continued their life cycle for all these centuries.

Nature, however, looks after all Her creatures, and the blue crab is no exception. When a male crab finds a female that is ready to take the big step in her life (just how he knows when the time is right is one of the great unsolved mysteries of the blue crab), he performs a mating dance that lets his future intended know exactly what he has in mind. If the female is interested she responds with some activity of her own. The whole thing ends with the male making a basket beneath him with his walking legs and carrying the submissive female within it. This is called a *cradle carry*, and will continue until the female busts out of her shell. It may take an hour, a day, or even a week or more, but come hell or high water, the male will not let "his woman" go once he has found her. When a male and female *in the cradle* are caught in traps or with scapping nets, they are called *doublers*.

Finally the big moment arrives. The female busts out of her shell and the two crabs get down to business, usually in shallow water and often under the protective cover of vegetation. This can last for a considerable length of time, possibly as long as 12 hours, making crabs one of the Don Juans of the undersea set, and

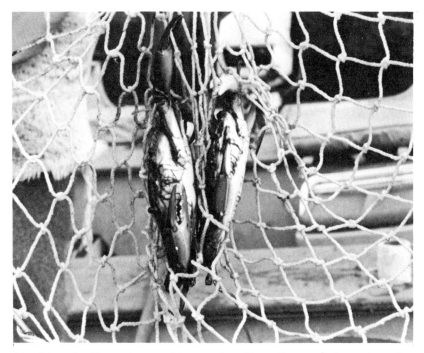

Doublers in the net, caught on a dropline; the male is on top, the female beneath him.

afterwards the gallant male again puts his partner in the cradle position. He will continue to carry the female until her shell has hardened and she is not helpless. Once they part, however, it is for keeps. The male may go on and mate several times during his life, but as for the lady, this was her one and only love affair. (Sorry, girls!)

Once the crabs have gone their separate ways, the females will usually begin heading toward the ocean, particularly if it is at the end of August or later. Certainly by mid-September in the northern and mid-Atlantic region, fertilized females are streaming toward the saltier waters of the sea in large numbers. Few will actually enter the ocean, however, preferring to spend the winter in the mud of deeper water at the mouths of estuaries and other places where the water has a higher salt content than that in which they spent the summer, since higher salinity content is necessary for egg hatching. Females do not have to immediately use the sperm they receive from the male; most crabs that mate in August or September will fertilize their eggs the following spring.

Depending on the weather, males and immature females will linger in shallow water for awhile longer after the mature female has departed. However, as the water and weather turns colder, these crabs too will begin heading for deeper depths. Finally, when the water hits about 40 degrees, the crabs will begin digging into the mud until nothing more than the tips of their eye stalks and their antennae are left sticking out of the bottom to indicate their presence. Once this happens, your crabbing season is over, although in reality as the crabs get into deeper water it becomes more difficult for the recreational crabber to reach them anyway. Crabs lie dormant in the mud throughout the cold weather, disturbed only by the giant commercial dredges that sweep across the bottom and rip them rudely out of their winter beds to take them to market.

The further south you go, however, the shorter the period of dormancy; everything depends on the temperature of the water and the weather. A general rule of thumb is that in the waters of Florida and the Gulf Coast, blue crabs tend not to bother with their mud beds during winter. Instead they just go through a lethargic period during which you might still be able to catch some, but they're certainly not going to be feeding with the intensity of summer.

It's said that in spring, a young man's fancy turns to love. Love, or at least the adventure of mating, is also on the mind of the female blue crab as well in spring, for she comes out of the mud and uses the sperm received from the male the previous year to fertilize her eggs. As the eggs develop, they form a large mass on the female's abdomen that resembles a sponge. Female crabs in this condition are commonly called *sponge crabs,* although they have many other colorful names, including berried crabs, busted sook, and cushion crabs.

Most states outlaw the taking of sponge blue crabs; some do not. If you catch a sponge crab, no matter whether it's legal or not to keep her, use some common sense and throw her back. If everyone kept sponge crabs, then eventually the species would cease to exist, and that hardly makes sense. Each crabber carries the responsibility for perpetuating the sport on his or her shoulders each and every time they go crabbing; don't blow it! Within the sponge sac females carry between 700,000 and two million eggs. It's a good thing this number is so high, because newly-hatched crabs face considerable obstacles to reach maturity. Estimates are that just one of every million eggs survives to become a market-sized adult blue crab.

As the crab moves about the water, the sponge sac ruptures and the eggs drift out, often initially clinging to the mother's legs or lower body. As the female travels, the eggs fall off. The mother, however, never looks back; her role in her offspring's lives is over, as is her own life. After releasing her eggs, the female crab usually dies. Hopefully, however, she has not died in vain. If the right conditions are present (temperature, water salinity, lack of predators, etc.) the eggs she has dropped hatch into microscopically-small crab larvae called *zoeas*.

If you could see zoeas milling about in the water (they have no means of swimming or self-locomotion, so milling pretty

Crab larva in the zoea stage.

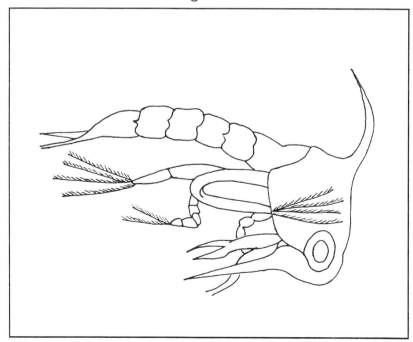

much sums up all they're capable of) you would never guess that you were looking at baby blue crabs. Zoeas resemble creatures from another planet in some cheap science fiction movie: they have incredibly large eyes, a fat body, a long pointed tail, and a single dorsal fin jutting up from their back.

Zoeas go through about eight moults. Each one slowly changes it into something that looks a bit more like a blue crab. Finally, after the eighth moult, the zoea becomes a *megalops*. This is the really big change in a crab's life. Now just large enough to be seen by a pair of sharp human eyes, the megalops has two small claws, its entire complement of walking legs, and the beginnings of its shell. Its eyes still look like something out of *It Conquered the World*, (in fact, megalops means "large eyes") and it still has a very un-crablike tail, but the similarity to what it will ultimately become is plainly evident.

Crab larva in the megalops stage.

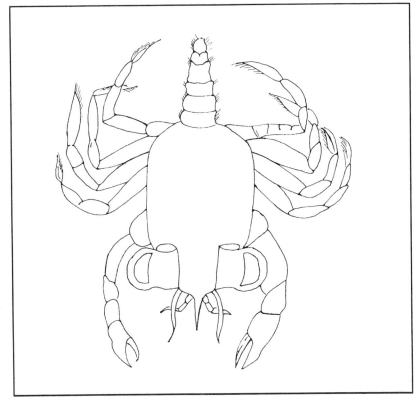

The megalops continues to moult, gradually losing its tail while increasing the width of its shell, until finally it truly resembles a blue crab for the first time. This entire sequence of events, from hatching to young blue crab, takes about two months. From this point on, the crab continues to exchange each shell for a progressively larger one until it's about an inch or two in length. This takes most of the summer, so that when cold winds and dropping water temperatures announce winter's approach, the young crab follows the example of its elders and slips into the mud. The following spring the young crabs come out of the mud and begin eating and moulting. By June they will have become about three inches long. From this point on they continue to grow by moulting, until they die of old age, get eaten by predators, or get caught (hopefully by you after reading this book). Three years is considered old in the crab kingdom; four years is ancient.

Moulting is, of course, how crabs grow. Females moult around 20 times during their life, while males go through it a few more times. As might be expected, the bigger a crab gets, the more time between moults. Although moulting is a fairly routine procedure for a crab when small, it grows progressively more difficult as the crab gets larger. It's during moulting that a crab's ability to casually sever a leg or claw comes in handy; uncooperative limbs can be left behind quickly and easily, although too much of this could well cause death. Some researchers speculate that moulting difficulties kill a good many older males that are wily enough to have escaped crabbers. Males moult until they die, while the ladies moult until they reach sexual maturity.

The process of moulting is fascinating to observe. A crab that sheds its shell is called a *softshell*, and is much prized by those who love seafood because you get to eat the crab without bothering to extract the meat from underneath the hard shell. (See Chapter 7 for more information on how to catch softshells).

Before a crab sheds, it often does two things: the first is that, several days prior to moulting, a crab eats like there is no tomorrow to store food up for the shedding phase, during and after which it does not eat at all. The second thing that a crab ready to moult does is head for shallow water, because that's where the vegetation it needs for protection is thickest. This is the reverse of usual, when a crab normally avoids shallow water because of the increased sunlight there.

Shedding its shell is an exhausting experience for the crab that leaves it weak and helpless. Gradually, after shedding it regains its strength, but until the new shell hardens, which normally takes a few days, the crab is still relatively easy pickings for any hungry predator that happens along. All it can do is hold up its claws threateningly and hope to bluff its way out of a tight spot. If the predator chooses to investigate further, however, the softshell crab is a dead duck.

When the crab is ready to shed, a crack appears at the base of its shell, between the two swimming paddles. The shell lifts up and the crab begins backing out of it. The more the crab backs out, the higher the broken shell rises up. When the crab is finally free it lies motionless behind its old shell, gathering its strength. People who are unfamiliar with crabs and stumble across such a sight often think there are two crabs present, so perfectly does the crab's new appearance match the old shell.

Once it is free, the crab begins taking in a lot of water. This helps it expand its muscles to fit its new, larger shell. Over the next few days the shell goes through the following phases as it hardens: papershell, tinback or buckram, and finally hardshell. When the crab is convinced that its shell will again protect it from its enemies it goes out and resumes eating. However, for awhile newly–shed crabs will have very little meat in them, and if you catch one, it makes sense to throw it back. If a crab feels light, and you suspect it might be a recent shedder, one sure way to tell is to look at the bottom of the crab: if it's bright white, or brighter than the others in your bushel basket, you've caught a recent shedder.

Now that you know all about how crabs go through their lives, it's time to put this knowledge to use and discover where to find these tasty shellfish.

Chapter Four
What Crabs Like, and Don't Like

It might seem obvious to state that if you knew something about the habits, life cycle, likes, and dislikes of the blue crab you would greatly increase your catch. Yet it's surprising how many recreational crabbers spend a lot of time and money (especially if they rent a boat) going after crabs where they simply are not likely to be found. While you don't have to have a Chesapeake bayman's instinctive knowledge of a crab's everyday habits, it does stand to reason that arming yourself with a bit of knowledge will help make your crabbing expeditions more enjoyable and your dinner table more laden with luscious blue crabs.

Since you aren't trying to make a living by catching blue

Everyone loves crabs.

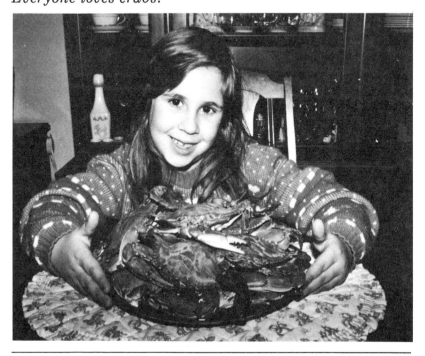

crabs, it isn't necessary to wade through a long recitation of everything ever known about crabs. However, there are several factors you should be aware of before heading out after these clever shellfish. The first, and most important, is: crabs are unpredictable. You can analyze, study, and observe them to death, and just when you think you've got them figured out, they'll do something completely opposite of what you think they're going to do. The moral is that crabs, like we humans, are subject to their own particular moods and whimsies. The day someone does totally figure out why a blue crab does what it does will be the day all the fun and suspense is taken out of crabbing. Thus, use the following information as a guideline, but don't take it to be written in stone. Once you think you've got a handle on crabbing, experiment a little bit; deviate from what this book says. Maybe someday you'll be writing a book about crabbing.

Weather/Temperature

The length of your crabbing season depends upon where you live. As stated in Chapter 3, when cold weather hits, crabs head for deeper water and bury themselves in the mud (although mature females begin heading for deeper water after they mate). Once crabs go into the mud, they are out of reach of the recreational crabber. Crabs neither moult nor eat when they are dormant. However, interestingly enough, research seems to indicate that dormant crabs act much like human sleepers: they toss, turn and move about in herky-jerky fashion.

What makes them "go into the mud" is a source of much speculation. It is generally agreed that once the water drops into the mid-50's, crabs leave the shallow areas they prefer and head for deeper water. Sometimes, the change can be quite startling; one day the crabs are still in the shallows, the next they're gone. Often a pronounced cold snap will sweep crabs out of the shallows like a broom; a major northwest storm, with its cold Canadian winds, can herald the crab's disappearance, especially in northern and mid-Atlantic states, where late summer/early autumn cold fronts often produce striking changes in the weather. Once the water drops to about 40 degrees, crabs know that winter has definitely arrived and will head for the mud.

What this means to you, the recreational crabber, is the following: If you live anywhere from Massachusetts to the Chesapeake Bay, your crabbing season will most likely run from May through mid-October. From the Chesapeake down to Florida, the water and air stay warmer longer, and so the season is generally from April through November. Florida and the Gulf Coast states normally provide year-round crabbing, although, as noted earlier, crabs in these waters go through a sluggish period.

If you're the type who waits impatiently for winter to end, scoop net in hand and pre-baited lines and traps sitting in your freezer, then the best thing for you to do is to keep track of the water temperature, not only where you live but also further south. The warmer the water is down south, the earlier the crabs will begin to stir and start trekking northward.

Keeping an eagle eye on the weather and water temperature is most critical in the early spring and early fall. Autumn especially is a tricky time, because one day the crabs can be running and the next they're gone. If you're not certain if the crabs are still there, call your favorite bait shop or boat rental dock and try to find out.

Types of Bait

Most people, knowing that blue crabs are scavengers, think that they will be attracted by any slimy, putrid piece of bait tossed at them. In fact, nothing could be more wrong. While it's true that crabs are scavengers – and even cannibals – they are picky scavengers. If they had noses, blue crabs would turn them up at the disgusting things that people try to entice them with. What they seem to prefer is bait that has just been thawed out – "fresh over ice," as it were. Even live bait doesn't seem to work as well as something that has just shaken off the chills from the freezer.

What does this mean for you? Normally, the same place you rent or dock your boat or someplace very close by will have all the bait you need. One of the most popular is a fish known as menhaden, which is often called "moss bunker" or just "bunker." Bunker is cheap and plentiful, and, since it's not too large, can be easily divided into sections. Fish heads work best for bait, because you can secure it easily by running string or wire through the eye sockets.

Another type of bait that seems to work fairly well is chicken. However, rest assured you're not going to have to serve Mr. Perdue's best; chicken remnants that cost just a few cents a pound, such as backs and necks, will do nicely for blue crabs.

Veteran crabbers and Maryland baymen who make their living off the blue crab often use salted eel as bait. This, however, can be expensive.

What makes the best crabbing bait is a topic that will be hotly argued until the end of time. Everyone has something that works best for them. A friend of mine used to swear by hot dogs as bait. For him they worked; on my line they just looked silly. The one constant in what type of fish works best is that oily fish, such as bunker, mackerel, bluefish, and eel, seems to work better than

Chicken parts make very good bait for crabs; other essentials are a sharp knife and strong string. The cooler in the background can be used for storing crabs, ice, or just some cold drinks.

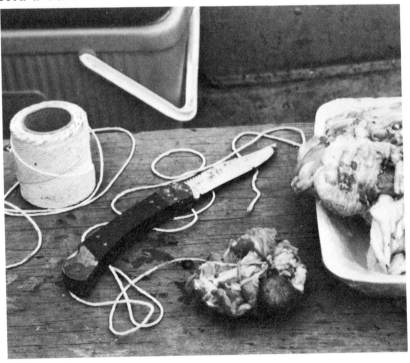

"non-oily." This could be because crabs are thought to have a keen sense of smell, and possibly the fish oil scent attracts them. Of course, this does not rule out using virtually any other type of fish or meat to attract crabs. Liver, meat scraps, any kind of fish, even animal bones with some meat on them – all can be tried and evaluated as crab bait. If something works for you, then stick with it – no matter how strange it may seem.

Water Conditions and Levels
This is where most recreational crabbers get tripped up. They think that simply because blue crabs usually live in salt water, they should be found in any body of salt water. But the reality is that crabs like a certain type of water, and certain water conditions. Furthermore, the time of year also has a lot to do with where blue crabs may be at any one particular time.

Sound confusing? It's really not. The key point to remember is that crabs like a mixture of salt and fresh water. This doesn't mean that you have to run around measuring the salinity of the water, unless you're so inclined; just use common sense and trial and error to figure out where the crabs are. In general, the further away from the ocean's influence you go in a body of water, the lesser the salinity of that water. Thus crabbing at the mouth of the bay, where it empties into the ocean, is not likely to be as productive as going further into the bay, where it is fed by fresh water streams or rivers. Tidal rivers and estuaries are normally bodies of water that provide excellent crabbing. While these names may sound strange to you, if you're at all familiar with bodies of water or the shore you've probably been on one or both of them.

A tidal river is, simply, a river where the water level fluctuates with high and low tides, just like the ocean. And just because they're called "rivers" doesn't mean something on the order of the Mississippi. Indeed, the best tidal river will be one that really shrinks down to almost nothing at extreme low tide. Yet, as long as there is some water flow to it then (evidence, more than likely, of fresh water feeder streams), that type of river should be a crabbing gold mine when the tide is changing (especially when it's coming in; see below).

An estuary is even easier to find. This is an "arm" of the sea, so to speak, that is still fed by the Atlantic's salt water. The Chesapeake Bay is an example of the perfect estuary for crabbing. Of course, having fresh water feed into the estuary is important, and will also often provide an easy way to enter the estuary via boat so you don't have to approach it from the ocean.

There are, however, exceptions to the salinity rule. As we discussed in Chapter 3, after females mate they usually begin heading for saltier water. If you can find their path and place yourself smack in the middle of it, you will reap a real bonanza of female crabs. This is also true in the early spring, when pregnant females awaken from their winter rest and seek a place to drop their eggs. At this time, if they haven't done so already, females will seek out water of a higher salinity, such as at or near the mouth of a bay, because once hatched zoeas need a high degree of salinity in order to survive.

Another important thing to remember about blue crab habitat is water depth. In general, depths of no more than 20 feet are desirable for crabbing. Anything deeper than that is not practical for recreational crabbers in several respects, not the least of which is that if you have to spend all day pulling up droplines and trap cords measuring 20 feet in length you're going to be one tired crabber at the end of the day!

When not moulting or at the end of the season, blue crabs prefer the shallow depths. I have been crabbing in just a few feet of water, where at extreme low tide you could look down and see the bottom, although this is not desirable because this means that crabs, with their excellent eyesight, can also look up and see you. But if you can find a depth of around 10 feet in a tidal river or estuary, with a supply of aquatic vegetation nearby, you're looking at ideal crabbing conditions.

You can judge where blue claws will be, depth-wise, by the time of year. From mid-spring and through the summer, crabs can be found at depths of between 10 to 30 feet. When feeding during this time, however, crabs are more likely to be in shallower water, something on the order of 6 to 10 feet. This is your best chance to catch them, because they're hungry and you're offering food. As the water and weather get colder, they go from depths of

30 feet all the way to depths of 60 to 80 feet. When they're moulting, you can find them in anything from a foot of water to around four or five feet.

Remember that crabs, like people and all other animals, have specific likes and dislikes. They enjoy waters where there is a good deal of bottom vegetation. They also have a penchant for old wood, which is why you see so many clinging to docks and pilings just below the surface of the water. If there are places in the water where a supply of waste food or fish is being tossed (not too likely in this day and age, but not everyone follows dumping laws strictly), then head there with all possible speed. There is nothing that crabs like better than snacking on human garbage. It is for this reason that a fishing pier sometimes offers superb crabbing, because the fishermen dump their leftover bait into the water and the crabs know it.

If all of this sounds a little bewildering, relax; it's not as hard as it seems. A few dollars invested in some tidal charts or even just general maps can help you find tidal rivers, estuaries, and depths very quickly. Another way is to ask around for the best spots, particularly at bait and boat shops. But you don't have to be a nautical genius, or spend hours poring over tidal charts, to find good crabbing spots. Just some basic observation of a river or bay will reveal what types of boats ride the waters there, and if people are out crabbing, fishing, etc.

Miscellaneous Likes and Dislikes
There are other factors to be considered when going after the wily blue crab. While none of these will make or break a crabbing trip, it's always nice to know as much as possible about your adversary. (It's also a way to appreciate the blue crab, an animal that, because of its looks and lousy disposition, has often been dismissed as a creature worthy of human respect.)

Crabs love to ride the tides. This has been an axiom of crabbing that has always worked for me. My grandfather used to only go crabbing either during or just before a full moon, because of the greater tidal pull that the full moon exerts. Experience has shown that the absolutely best times to be waiting for crabs is when high tide is coming in, and when it is heading out.

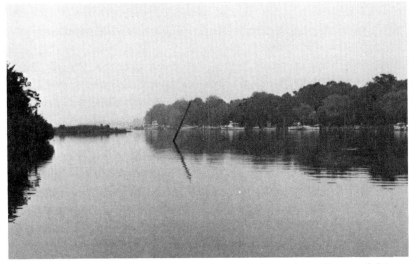

This quiet, backwater lagoon is a perfect place for crabbing.

Crabs like slow-moving waters. Dropping your lines or traps into a swiftly-flowing current is not likely to gain you too many crabs. Blue crabs are perpetual roamers, who like to meander over a wide area while they seek to satisfy their voracious appetite. A rapid current doesn't allow them the freedom to do this because it acts like an invisible hand, hurrying the crab along. It is also much harder to control lines and traps in water that moves swiftly.

Crabs dislike sunlight. They are the vampires of the underwater world. The surest way to lose a crab off a dropline is to bring it up too close to the surface, so that it feels or sees the rays of the sun. This is why the best time to go crabbing is very early morning, before the sun has climbed too high, or later in the afternoon, when it is sinking in the western sky. Mid-day – when the sun is directly overhead and throwing its light straight into the water below – has always been one of the worst times to crab. An added bonus of crabbing during the late afternoon is that this time of day often brings out big males, especially during mating season. Although it may bring instant bags to your eyes, the absolutely best time to go crabbing is very early in the morning, around five o'clock or so.

Crabs dislike noise, or sudden movement. Since their eyesight is so keen, it doesn't take much to make a blue crab flash away from your line. A lot of waving or other gyrations when you're pulling up a dropline is not recommended. Noise, such as that coming from a portable boom-box in your boat, is also not a good idea. Remember, crabs are used to scooting along the bottom in relative calm, seeking out food and/or mates in obscurity. They're not likely to patronize a boat that sounds like the Playboy Mansion at party time.

Now that you know what crabs like, and what they don't like, it's time to get serious. Put on your game face, because next we're going to discuss precisely how to catch the often-elusive blue crab.

Chapter Five
Catching the Elusive Blue Crab

Now we come to the heart of the matter – catching the blue crab. Many people think that catching crabs is easy; crabs are not very intelligent, they reason, so how hard could it be? These are the same people who usually have a paltry half-dozen or so crabs in their bushel basket after a long day's work.

Truthfully, crabbing is not hard. In fact, it's one of the most enjoyable water-based recreational activities around. And those people mentioned above were right: crabs are not smart. It's quite common to pull a dropline all the way out of the water and have a baby blue crab still clinging tenaciously to the bait. (Undoubtedly the adults on the bottom shake their antennae in dismay at this sorry spectacle, but when was the last time that kids listened to grown-ups anyway?)

But don't be fooled. Crabs are clever and resourceful. Their skittishness, combined with amazing quickness and excellent eyesight, makes crabbing one of the most challenging of all sports – and that much more rewarding when done successfully.

Before talking about how to catch them, however, there are a couple of important points to cover. The first is how to measure a crab, or when you know a crab is a *keeper*. Blue crabs are measured tip-to-tip, which is sometimes referred to as point-to-point. The tips of a blue crab are the last two protruding points of the shell, which are located in the rear, one on each side. A crab is measured from the outside of one tip to the outside of the other. If this distance measures five inches, then the crab is considered a five-incher, no matter what the dimensions are of the rest of the shell. Unless you're the type who can determine an accurate measurement with just a glance, it's always a good idea to bring a ruler or tape measure along with you on a crabbing trip. Anything that measures within the legal size limit is a *keeper;* others should be thrown back.

While we're on the subject of legal size limits, you should check with your local fish and/or wildlife office to find out what the regulations are for blue crab crabbing in your state or area. Crabbing regulations can be incredibly complex. It was originally my intention to include an easy-to-read chart of some simple crabbing rules for each state in this book, but I soon abandoned the idea when I realized that the words "simple" and "crabbing rules" are mutually exclusive! For example, in some states you have to be a resident to legally crab; in others, you don't; in Massachusetts, you have to be a property owner. Some states have restrictions on taking sponge crabs; some don't. Some states have restrictions on what type of equipment you can use; some don't. Many states have different descriptions of what constitutes a keeper. Do you see what I mean by "complex?" To save yourself a lot of headaches afterwards, do some checking on the regulations and laws beforehand.

Droplines

Droplines (also called "handlines") are probably the oldest method of crabbing in history. It's easy to picture a prehistoric man waving good-bye to his wife and kiddies in the cave and then heading out to a nearby river with a fish head attached to a long, thick vine, ready to spend the day catching crabs for dinner.

But, as is often the case, the old ways are the best ways. Absolutely nothing beats the challenge and thrill of dropline crabbing. The odds against you are great, to be sure; one false move – one inadvertent jerk of the line, a miscue with the net, a sudden flash of sunlight – and that luscious six-inch blue crab that was chomping happily on your bait a moment ago will vanish. The frustration of having a big one drop off your line at the last possible moment can only be compared to when your ten-year-old child tells you at breakfast that she has a major science project due that day for school that she hasn't started yet.

Droplines sum up what sport is supposed to be all about: just you versus the prey. It's wile and guile against instinct and survival.

What's nice about droplines is that they're simple. All you need is a good, sturdy piece of twine, although any heavy string

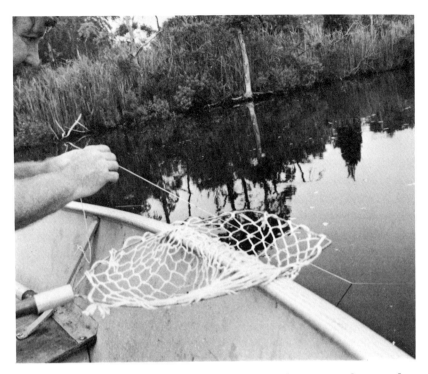

Pulling in a dropline from a boat, with net at the ready.

will do just fine as long as it absorbs water and sinks. (Some strings and twines are very porous, and tend to float, particularly those that contain a lot of plastic.) Although you can buy special "crabbing line," any type of thick string or twine is just as good, and probably cheaper.

Another good thing about droplines is that you can use them almost anywhere: a pier, a dock, a boat, or the shore. Using droplines on a boat is sometimes difficult, because the boat's continual rocking motion may occasionally scare a crab away. A swell from a passing boat, strong tidal movements, or the briskness of the afternoon sea breeze may also cause crabs to prematurely bolt. However, once you get the hang of it, droplining from a boat is a lot of fun.

There's no great scientific principle behind droplining; it's easy and simple to learn. Just tie one end of your line to a piece of bait. Secure the other end to something permanent, like a nail, oar lock, piling, etc., then toss the bait into the water. The bait should be heavy enough to sink to the bottom, since that's where crabs spend most of their time. If the current is strong enough to pull the bait, and it winds up streaming out in the water like an undersea pennant, use a small sinker to weight the line down. Remember to tie the bait tight – very tight – and check it after it's been in the water for awhile. This is particularly important for bait that was frozen when you first threw it in the water; as it thaws out it will contract, and the knot will loosen. Once the line is in the water, the waiting game begins. Crabs need time to find your bait, and it's almost guaranteed they won't come near it if you're pulling the line up every ten seconds and throwing it back again with a loud splash. Constant movement disturbs both the bottom and the surface of the water, and causes crabs to stay away. The main thing to learn about droplining is patience, patience, patience. If you're the type who fidgets at the movies, use another crabbing method. The most productive lines are those that are checked every few minutes, at the very least.

When the time does come to check your line, grasp it gently between your thumb and forefinger and pull it towards you ever so slightly. If there's a slight resistance and/or vibration, it's likely there's a crab on the other end. It is impossible to describe what it feels like when there's a crab on a dropline; even the most skilled crabbers get fooled and think that they have a crab, only to pull the line in and find nothing. The longer you use droplines, the more familiar you'll be with the feeling. The best way to explain it is that, when a crab's present, it's almost as if the line has a pulse.

Droplines should always be brought in slowly, especially if you're fortunate enough to have a blue crab on the other end. The object is to bring the line up without knocking the crab off. Remember, there's nothing holding the crab to your line except its appetite, and if you make it too difficult, the blue claw will decide to forget the whole thing and look for a less bothersome source of food.

At first, as you gather up the excess line, the bait will move across the bottom and it won't be too hard for the crab to stay with it. But at some point the bait is going to leave the bottom and

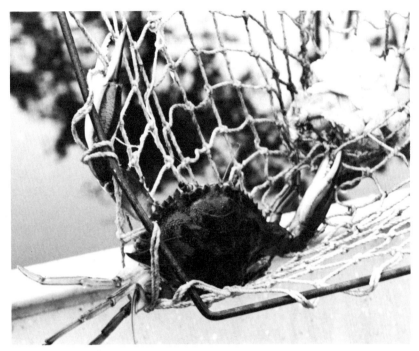

What all crabbers hope to see – a delicious blue crab in their scoop net.

come up through the water toward the surface – and you. That's why you want to use the delicate touch of a surgeon when pulling in the line.

As you work the line in take your long handled net – commonly called a dip net or scoop net and slip it into the water close to where the bait, and hopefully the crab, will appear on its trip up from the bottom. It's important that the net be put into the water gently; a splash or other movement will send the crab scurrying away. Make sure that the net is deep enough in the water so that you can bring it up smoothly and swiftly underneath or behind the crab, but shallow enough so that you can see it and control its action (hence the need for a long handle).

The moment that the bait has been brought up far enough so you can see the crab hanging onto it, bring the net over the crab as quickly as possible. Some people advocate pulling the bait right up to the surface before they scoop, but this is risky business. A crab has excellent eyesight, and the better you can see it, the better it can see you. It's far better to bring the net up from below the crab while it's still feeling somewhat secure in the water and occupied with your bait. As soon as you net the crab, try to pull the baited line out of the net. Doing this will eliminate the need to battle the crab for the bait, because once it's been netted and hoisted out of the water, a crab will inevitably cling to the bait like a nervous bride to her father. Trying to disengage one from the other (the crab from the bait, not the bride from her father) can be a tedious task. Once you have the crab netted just flip it into your basket.

That's all there is to droplining. It actually sounds more complicated than it is. Remember the four basic rules of droplining:

1. Keep the line as steady as possible.
2. If the current is strong, use a sinker to weight the line down so it lays on the bottom.
3. Bring the line up slowly.
4. Have a scoop net ready to net the crab once the bait comes into view.

Droplines will work well off a beach too. Here the situation is a little different, because you're pulling the bait toward you along the ground, and not up through the water. However, the principle is the same, except that you'll be bringing the net from behind the crab, rather than underneath it. To use droplines from a beach, just tie the line around something that can be pushed firmly into the ground, such as a wooden stake or pole. Attach your line to the pole, then set it in the water a few feet from the shoreline and cast your line into the deeper water. The same rules about bringing the crab along slowly apply here as well. It's also important that you wade into the water at least up to where the stake is secured when you're ready to net the crab, because the crab is going to be extremely aware that it's being moved into shallow water, so the further out you can go the better your chances of netting it before it bolts.

Once you decide that you like the challenge of droplining, you can do it from almost anywhere. It truly is one of the purest forms of sport around!

Crab Traps

Crab traps, also called handtraps or crab baskets, are the "next step" for the recreational crabber. You can catch more crabs with less effort with traps than with lines, but the challenge isn't the same. However, for people who either can't or won't bother with droplines, traps are an excellent alternative.

Essentially a wire box with four sides that open and close, crab traps can be purchased at any sporting goods store, department store, or fishing/hunting store. The way a trap works is simple: it sits on the bottom with a piece of bait tied in the middle and all four sides open. When you pull the main line – known as the control line – that feeds up to the surface, the four sides slam shut, trapping the crab inside.

Normally crab traps are purchased unassembled, but they're easier to put together than most kids' toys. The important thing to remember is to make certain that the lines attached to each side that feed into the control line are the same length, so that when the control line is pulled, each side closes tightly. Crabs can

A crab trap all baited and ready to go. It should look just like this, with all four sides open, when it rests on the bottom

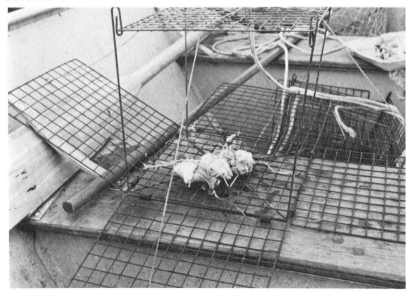

escape very easily from a trap that does not slam shut like a jail cell door.

Another place where beginning crabbers get "trapped" by traps is that they don't use heavy enough line, so when they pull the trap up they feel a sudden snap, and the line breaks. This leaves your trap sitting peacefully on the bottom, where it will undoubtedly serve as a risk-free crab restaurant until your bait is gone. Use thick twine, heavy string, or something similar – my grandfather used rope, and I still do – or be prepared to pay the consequences.

Since traps require all four sides to be open to work properly,

Doublers caught in a trap.

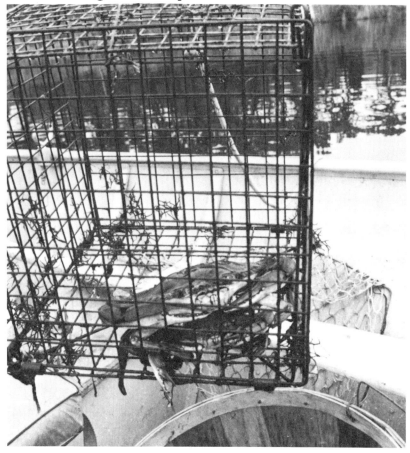

they are only effective on flat bottoms. Areas that contain rocks, thick vegetation, or a large amount of bottom debris are not good locations for traps. And, like lines, traps work best when left alone for a time. In fact, leaving traps undisturbed might be even more critical, because they cause a considerable commotion when pulled up and tossed back into the water. It takes time for everything to settle down once a trap hits the bottom; crabs need time as well to overcome their reluctance to approach anything that causes a lot of discord.

Traps come in several different designs, including so-called star or triangle traps, which have three sides that close instead of four. Experiment with both types until you find one you like. The basic rules of using crab traps are:

1. Tie the bait securely on the bottom center panel of the trap.
2. Make sure that when the control line is played out, all four sides open completely and lie flat.
3. Use traps only in areas where the bottom is flat and smooth.
4. Pull the control line hard; this should slam shut the four sides and trap the crab inside. If this does not happen, adjust the lines from each side until you get a tight fit.

Scapping

If you thought droplining was easy, wait until you try scapping. You don't even need bait!

Scapping is just a crabbing term for catching crabs using a long-handled net. Although some people make scapping seem like some mystical experience, all it really means is walking around with your crabbing net and snagging crabs that you happen to see. Scapping can also be done in a boat, by poling gently through the shallows and keeping a wary eye out for crabs on the bottom.

One of the best places to scap for crabs is on the pilings of docks, piers, or other structures with a foundation below the surface of the water. For some unknown reason, crabs love to hang onto wood, the older and more decrepit the better. An old barnacle-encrusted railroad trestle near where I live attracts flocks of blue crabs. Thus you can often see a nice-sized blue crab clinging onto a dock piling just below the surface of the water, seemingly oblivious to all else in the world.

Notice, however, that I said "seemingly." Those same attributes – sharp eyesight, quickness, and sideways swimming ability – that serve the blue crab so well in other cases also come into play here. If you expect to just plunge your net into the water and snag a crab off of a piling, forget it; it'll be gone before the mesh is barely wet. To be a successful scapper, you must use those same attributes that served *you* so well during droplining: quickness, reflexes, and sneakiness.

The first thing to do is try and anticipate the crab's likely escape route when it sees or senses the net coming toward it. Be prepared to move the net that way instantly, although also be ready to jerk it the other way if the crab does something unexpected. Next, try to have the net in the water and moving toward the crab as soon as possible. This will help you not only gain an element of surprise, but will also enable you to better gauge how much your final lunge at the crab will be slowed by water resistance.

That's really all there is to scapping: find crab, sneak up on crab, and try to catch crab before it zips away.

As mentioned above, any type of old wood acts as a crab magnet. Other places that work well are areas where fishermen traditionally throw left-over bait into the water, or other places where human food refuse is plentiful.

You can also scap by wandering through the shallows, particularly along cattail-choked streams where most boats can't even go. Crabs – and here's another exception to those crabbing rules – sometimes enjoy taking a piece of food and wandering almost up to the beach to enjoy a quiet meal. If you're stealthy, you can sometimes come upon them just sitting in no more than a few inches of water, eating away.

To become a skilled scapper, you have to find out where the crabs go, then work on your technique until you catch more than you let get away. Some will always get away; even the greatest scappers blow it every once in a while. But with a little luck and some practice, you can soon be bringing home a decent catch of blue crabs by only using your trusty net.

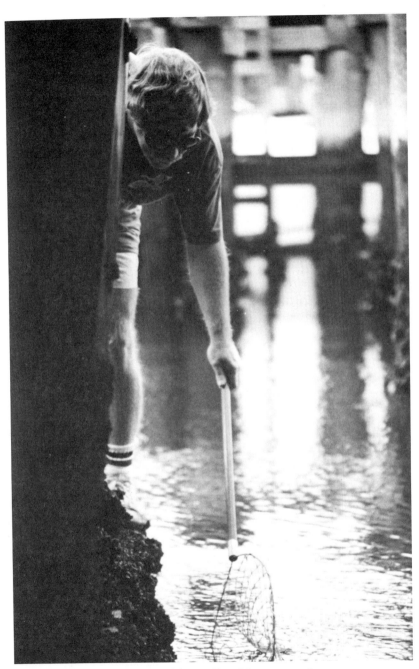

The scapper spots something, dips his net, and . . .

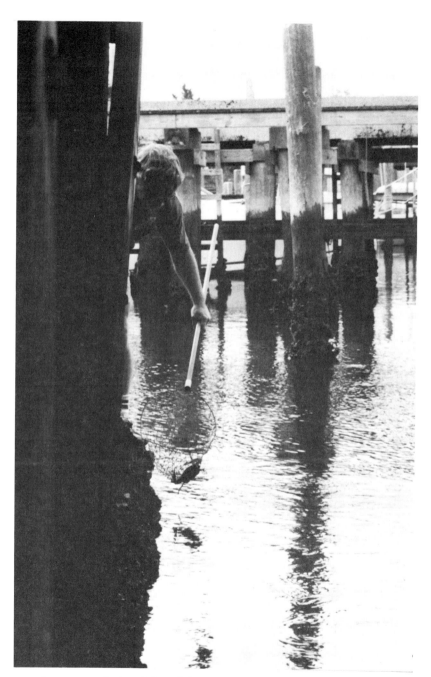

. . . is rewarded with a blue crab for his effort.

Night Crabbing

Night crabbing is sometimes called night scapping, and with good reason; the object – catching crabs without bait, using only a net – is the same.

Crabs are attracted to light. Why this is no one knows, but shining a big pool of light onto the water is like putting out a "come and get it" sign to blue crabs.

The most effective night crabbing is done from a boat, although the technique can also be practiced from the shoreline. Simply shine a powerful flashlight or other strong source of light on the water, and more often than not, a nice-sized crab will soon swim over to see what's going on.

Night crabbing works well because crabs tend to swim on the surface of the water at night, after the hated sunlight has disappeared. Experience has shown that many bigger crabs – particularly males – head for the shallows at night, possibly to look for mates. But you can also night crab by grabbing blue crabs off the bottom. Again, aiming a strong light through the water will both attract crabs, and help you see those that are scuttling right along.

Night crabbing in a boat usually requires at least two people: one to hold the light and pole the boat, the other to scap the crabs. Since navigating a boat at night is tricky, it's not recommended that you try it with less than two people. On the shore, however, you can easily night crab all by yourself.

If you find that you like night crabbing, you might want to get elaborate and build a more powerful light. Some veteran crabbers who go night scapping by boat use a mini-spotlight powered by a car battery. The more powerful the light, the more crabs it will attract. However, just a good, strong, "lantern-type" flashlight will make night crabbing an extremely enjoyable way to spend an evening.

Seining

Seining is another "baitless" way to catch crabs. This method, however, takes two people and a considerable bit of energy. A seining net is a long (approximately 20 feet), fine-mesh net attached to two long poles. There are sinkers along the bottom of the net, and floats across the top.

Each person grabs a pole, spreads out the net, wades into the water, then lets the net drop to the bottom. The sinkers pull the net down, while the floats prevent the top from dropping below the surface. The two people then drag the net across the bottom and toward the shore, catching whatever is in its path. This "sweep" continues until you reach the beach. The trick with seining is to make sure that each end pole scraps along the bottom; this makes the net itself pull across the bottom, which prevents anything from slipping underneath it and escaping.

As mentioned, it takes a lot of energy to seine, because you're pulling the net through the water at a fairly rapid clip, and water can be surprisingly heavy! But when you get the net on shore, it's always great fun to see exactly what you've caught. Quite often there are both hard and softshell crabs in the net, along with a variety of small fish such as killies that were in the wrong place at the wrong time when you came through with your seining net. Because seining requires you to wade out further in the water than you normally would, be sure to wear something on your feet so hidden rocks, broken glass or metal, or even crabs don't wind up making a painful impression on your tender pink foot (or feet).

Trotlines

The five crabbing methods just listed are common ones for recreational crabbers. The advantage with them is that they're basically simple, and can be used at a variety of locations at very little cost or trouble.

Trotlining is for the advanced crabber – someone who truly loves crabbing and wants to significantly increase his/her catch. The potential for catching dozens – even hundreds – of crabs by trotlining is very real. In fact, before crab pots, commercial crabbers used trotlines. The only flaw is that you need a boat. We will briefly talk about both trotlines and its commercial successor, crab pots, although they are really not methods usually employed by beginning or even casual crabbers.

A trotline is an ordinary thick twine or heavy cord line that ranges in length from several hundred to several thousand feet. (Beginners, however, are strongly recommended to stick to a "short" length of around 100 feet.) Every few feet pieces of bait are tied to the line. A trotline is meant to lay on the bottom of the water; in order to keep it in place (and also so you know where the line is located), the trotline is anchored at both ends, most often by cinder blocks or other heavy objects that will hold their ground against tidal flow. However, the trotline itself is not attached directly to the anchors; that would make it nearly impossible to pick up. Rather, the end of each trotline is attached to a float, which in turn is connected to an anchor.

Sound complicated? It really isn't. Just think of a trotline as one long submerged dropline, with a lot of pieces of bait attached. After the trotline has been laid on the bottom, the crabber positions his or her boat at one end of the trotline and begins moving the boat along the line, pulling the line up at the same time. As each "bait station" comes near the surface, the crab hanging onto the bait is scapped with a normal long-handled scoop net, just as is done with a dropline. As soon as the crabber is finished with one bait station the next one should be coming up, ready to be checked. In this way a crabber who runs several trotlines keeps constantly busy, and also nets a considerable number of blue crabs in the bargain.

If you decide that blue claw crabbing is your life, and you want to try running a trotline, here are a few hints: 1) To assure that the ends of the trotline (that which lead from the float) remain on the bottom, use a length of chain or other heavy object; 2) Because the crabs will be feeding on your bait for a much longer period of time, use "tough" bait, such as fish heads or eel, that can be tied very securely and won't be torn to bits by the time you reach each bait station; 3) Work the trotline by going with the tide – not against it; 4) Use a small, open boat like a rowboat, in order to give yourself the most maneuvering ability, both with the line and the net.

Crab Pots
Just as trotlining is for the advanced recreational crabber, crab pots are strictly for those people who don't want to "go" crabbing, but rather, just want to catch and eat crabs. But while trotlines take some skill, there is no challenge or sport with crab pots; they are merely instruments for pulling in large loads of

crabs. In many respects a crab pot is like a trap: you bait it, drop it into the water until it reaches the bottom, and then pull it up. For this reason crab pots are the method used by most commercial crabbers. As much as they'd probably enjoy sitting out on the water crabbing with a few droplines, commercial crabbers need to pull in all the crabs they can as often as possible, or they'd be out of business. This is why most commercial crabbers run several dozen – or even several hundred – pots at one time.

Crab pots require no participation on your part. After you bait the pot and put it into the water, you forget about it. Later that day, or even the next day, you pull the pot up and empty out your catch. The bait is put into a special compartment that lets the crabs see it and smell it, but not get to it (unlike a trap.) Once the crab goes into the pot, it almost never finds its way out. Eventually it gives up trying.

Like trotlines, crab pots are marked by lines attached to floats. Unfortunately, what sometimes happens is that unscrupulous people know what these floats mean, and will pull up the pots if the crabber is not around.

There are both commercial crab pots and "sport" crab pots on the market. If you decide to go this route, check over each type carefully. Remember that since crab pots stay in the water for hours at a time, they tend to rust and deteriorate rather quickly, so getting a sturdy, well-built pot is probably your chief consideration. If the cost of the pot is too great (it can run to $50 or more), try chipping in with a few friends. As long as someone has a boat, and you have a spot to drop the pot, it might be worth the money. When full of crabs, crab pots can be real heavy to pull up – maybe weighing as much as 35 pounds. (Commercial crabbers commonly use winches or other machines to pull up their pots.) Keep this in mind too before deciding to give crab pots a try.

Let's assume that you've chosen one of these crabbing methods. You went out one day, and were blessed with a fair wind, a calm sea, and dozens of hungry blue crabs clamoring to taste your bait. The crabbing has been so hot that steam rises from your scoop net every time you dip it into the water. Now what?

Chapter Six

Keeping Crabs Cool & Comfortable

So now you've done it – you've caught the elusive blue crab. In fact, not only have you caught this wily creature, but a whole bunch of its friends too. But it's too early to go back home; the day is young, and there are still crabs to be caught! So what do you do with the ones you've got?

Surprisingly, this seemingly simple question is something that trips up more recreational crabbers than anything else. Most people can figure out how to put a piece of bait on the end of a string and toss it into the water, but doing something intelligent and reasonable with their crabs after they have been caught is quite another story.

Where most people go wrong is in one of two ways: either they think that crabs survive just fine out of the water and in the broiling sun for several hours, or they feel that since crabs like water, they'll love being jammed into a small bucket of water along with dozens of other crabs. Unfortunately, without the proper guidance, both of these actions often lead to one thing: dead crabs by the time they are brought home.

The problem with dead crabs is the same as with all shellfish that expire before you put them into the pot: are they safe to eat? Some crabbers argue that you can safely cook and eat dead crabs within a few hours of their demise as long as you keep them cold; but this runs into the problem of exactly when is the magic line between safe and not safe crossed? Is a crab that died three hours ago not safe to eat, but one that died two hours ago is? And are you certain that it was just two hours ago? Maybe it was three, and the other one died four hours ago. And just how cold is cold?

My grandfather, who was the inspiration for this book and who forgot more about crabbing than I'll ever know, had a hard and fast rule about crabbing: you don't eat anything that isn't alive when you toss it into the pot. No if's, and's, or but's about it. His philosophy was that it just wasn't worth taking a chance, and that has always seemed like sound advice to me. There's another side to this whole issue as well. It is simply criminal to catch something just to let it die without eating it. Catching anything only to let it die is a crime against Nature. The way to avoid this whole dilemma, of course, is to not let your crabs expire before you get them home. A little thought and advance planning can help you do this, and also make sure that those delicious blue crabs you worked so hard to catch will make it into your mouth and not the garbage can.

I can't recall how many times I've seen people clamber out of a boat with a bushel basket full of crabs. The ones on top are dry and listless, their shells already turning white from over-exposure to the sun. It's a good bet that 25 percent, if not half, of these crabs might be dead by the time the people get them home and are ready to cook them.

Bushel baskets are every crabber's favorite way of carrying their catch, and they do have several advantages: they're light, easily picked up by the wire handles on both sides, and large enough to hold a good day's worth of blue crabs. However, they have one big disadvantage; they allow crabs to dry out quickly. A bushel basket sitting on the bottom of a rowboat for six hours under the withering mid-July sun must feel like an inferno to the crabs inside.

There are several very simple ways to keep crabs in bushel baskets from suffering this fate. The easiest is to keep something cool and wet over the crabs. This can be anything from a burlap bag to an old sheet; in an emergency it can even be done with newspaper, although the wetter a newspaper gets the more it deteriorates, which results in large chunks of wet newspaper mixing in with your crabs. The main thing to remember is to keep this "crab canopy" wet by continually dipping it into the water.

Another method for keeping your blue crabs wet, happy, and alive when you're in a boat is to periodically (and carefully) lean over the side and dip the bushel basket into the water. Since the sides are not sealed the water can easily rush in between the slats to give your crabs a refreshing shower. However, by doing this you will make the basket very heavy, at least until the water drains out, and if the bottom is a little weak, you could suddenly find yourself holding an empty basket while your crabs are swimming off (undoubtedly giggling) in all directions. If you're crabbing off a beach or in the shallows, you can put a heavy object in the bottom of the bushel basket to anchor it and leave the basket just beyond the water line, so that the ebb and flow of the water streams in and out of it. If you choose this method, just remember to keep an eye on the basket so that it doesn't get swept out to deeper water by the rising tide or a large swell from a passing boat.

Another common mistake recreational crabbers make is to have a plastic or metal bucket full of water, which they then proceed to fill with crabs. The problem here is that unless the water is changed frequently, the oxygen in it gets used up, and the crabs will die as surely as if they were left in a dry bushel basket. (If anybody ever figures out how to change the water in these buckets and not lose all their crabs in the bargain, let me know.)

Good storage receptacles for crabs are any type of heavy sack, such as those used to store 50 pounds of potatoes or onions, that are porous enough to enable water to pass through. Some people even submerge this type of sack in water, with their crabs inside. This becomes a bit tricky, however, when you have to put another crab into it, and you have to untie the knot at the top of the sack that keeps the crabs trapped inside. Trying to maneuver a scoop net containing a crab, while untying a knot in a sack full of more crabs, is quite a feat!

Some crabbers ignore both the bushel basket and the bucket and keep their crabs in large coolers filled with ice. This has the advantage of slowing crabs down somewhat, so that when you go to transfer them from container to pot they're not quite so feisty. However, it also means that you have to have a continuing source of fresh ice to replace that which melts.

In general, the faithful bushel basket is the best storage container for crabs. Just remember to keep the blue crabs wet and out of the direct sun. Keep in mind that you should never, ever, mix softshell and hardshell crabs. Hardshell crabs will attack their softshelled cousins unmercifully and, if you combine the two, by the end of the day you'll have only hardshells left.

Another thing that recreational crabbers have to learn is how to handle – pick up with your bare hands – crabs. I know that this sounds like something you'll never have to do (after all, you have a net, haven't you?) but take my word for it, at some point in your crabbing career the time will come when you're going to have to reach down and pick one of the little critters up. Since it's better if this is done without your knees knocking and nervous sweat pouring down your face, let's talk about exactly how you accomplish this. It really is easy, and with time and practice will come confidence, until before you know it you'll be ready to juggle live crabs on-stage at Las Vegas. (Well, that might be pushing it a bit!)

From the moment you catch a crab it begins trying to escape, whether it's from a scoop net or a storage bucket. In fact, the more crabs you catch, the greater the odds are that a Great Escape will occur. Crabs would have made great circus performers, because they're constantly standing on each other and straining vertically upward to reach the lip of the bushel basket or storage container they're in. So what do you do when you're in a small, confined space such as a rowboat, and suddenly hear a mad scuttling of legs and claws that makes you realize that one – or more – of your formerly captive crabs are now roaming around free on the bottom of the boat?

The first thing to remember is not to panic. Unless the crab is in a really bad mood, it's not going to rush up and attack you. The crab is looking for a hiding spot, and is as frightened of you as you are of it. However, having said that, remember that blue crabs are fearless fighters that do not retreat into their shells like turtles when cornered; if a crab is trapped it will gladly fight.

Blue crabs are as quick out of the water as they are in it. Try waving your hand over a bushel of crabs some time and watch how fast their claws spring up. Remember also that crabs have excellent eyesight. This means that you simply can't just "sneak up" on a crab, or rely on what some might suppose to be a human's superior quickness to grab a loose crab. If you do you'll almost certainly get your fingers nipped for the trouble, and once a blue crab has hold of something it takes an awful lot to make it let go. While the bite of a blue crab's claws won't kill you, it can cause a deep, painful cut.

A note of caution: if you are ever unfortunate enough to have a blue crab – or any other large crab – latch onto your finger with its claw, breaking the claw off from the crab's body will only make the pain worse. Why? Because crab claws spasmodically tighten just before they are broken off. The best way to remove a crab from your finger is to immerse it and the crab in a bucket of water, which will usually cause the crab to relax its grip.

The only safe place to handle a blue crab is in the back. Try envisioning an imaginary line that runs from between the crab's eyes to the very back of its shell, in the middle of its two swimming paddles; this is where you can grab a crab and not run the risk of having one of its claws find your finger. To do this safely, you must have the crab immobilized, or at least know that it can't suddenly whirl around and face you. The best way to stop a crab from moving is to keep your foot firmly on it. This is one reason why it's usually a good idea to wear some type of shoes during crabbing; old sneakers work well. Whatever you use,

One way to successfully hold a blue crab; the back legs as well as the back part of the shell are being held.

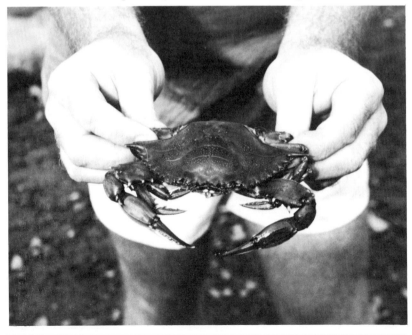

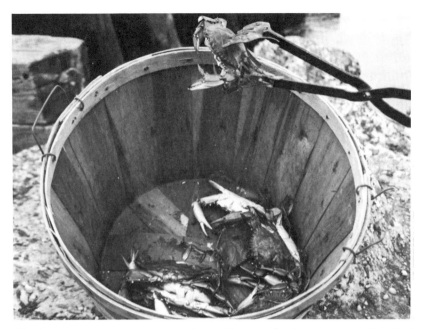

Crab tongs have many uses; handling crabs in and out of bushel baskets is only one of them.

however, don't crack the shell; you'd be surprised how easily your foot or some other heavy object can break a crab's shell.

When you grab a crab in the back, keep your thumb on top, your forefinger on the bottom, and the remaining three fingers tucked inside your palm. If you let your fingers stray too far underneath the crab, you're going to feel the sting of its claws. When you pick it up the crab will probably wave its claws, and possibly even its legs, but don't let that spook you; just keep a firm grip on it and return it to the storage container.

You can also hold a crab just above its back two appendages, which are the swimming paddles. If you grasp both the shell and the end of the swimming paddles, you won't put as much stress on the appendages. Again, however, remember to fold up the fingers you're not using.

However, for those people (guys and girls) who just won't pick up a crab, even if it's commandeering the oars and taking over the boat, there is another solution. Most bait and boat shops, and even department stores in crabbing regions, sell long-handled tongs that are perfect for picking up crabs from a safe distance away. Tongs like these also come in handy when it's time to wash the crabs off before cooking them.

Let's assume that everything on your crabbing trip has turned out okay. You caught a respectable amount of crabs, none of them got away (and if some did, there are no cut or bleeding fingers or toes), and they are all still alive.

But wait a minute! You're not going home just yet, are you? After all, there are still softshells to catch!

Chapter Seven
Seeking Out Softshells

As discussed in Chapter 3, when a crab sheds its shell it's called a softshell until the new shell hardens, which usually takes a few days. Softshell crabs are greatly sought after, both for their taste and for the fact that you can eat them shell and all. For many people, this beats prying off a crab shell any day!

Catching softshells, however, requires an entirely different set of tactics from hardshell crabbing. Softshells are neither plentiful nor easy to catch, which is why they cost so much at restaurants and seafood stores. However, if you can catch hardshells you can catch softshells; all it takes is a little patience and some knowledge of the blue crab's habits.

When crabs are ready to shed, they commonly come into shallow water, where the increased sunlight causes thicker vegetation to grow. A thick mat of vegetation, such as eelgrass provides, offers a tempting hiding place for *peelers* (crabs that are just about ready to moult). However, if neither eelgrass or thick vegetation is present in your crabbing location, don't despair; crabs that are ready to shed will seek out any type of shelter in the shallows. A collection of rocks, a pile of discarded building material such as cinder blocks . . . anything that makes the crab feel safe might be a softshell haven.

Because shedders come into shallow water, and you have to wade into the water in order to find them as well as locate vegetation beds that might be hidden during high tide, most softshell crabbing is done during low tide. It's a good idea to wear shoes when seeking softshells, since you often will not be able to see where you're stepping.

You catch softshells by lurking quietly around the shallows with your scoop net, looking for any crabs sitting on the bottom. Sometimes, if you come across a crab that has just moulted, it will be sitting directly behind its discarded shell, giving the

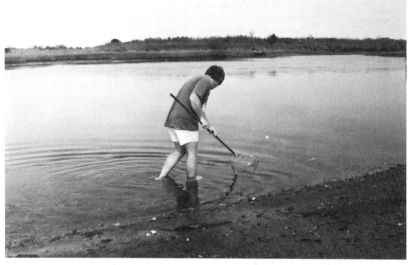
Looking for softshells in shallow water.

appearance of two crabs. Don't be fooled! Go for the one in the rear with your net. Sometimes, veteran crabbers will comb through vegetation beds with their nets even if they don't see a crab, figuring that a peeler might likely be hiding there. You can try this too, although be prepared to really force your net through the vegetation; eelgrass is especially thick. In some fishing/boating stores you can buy a special softshell net for this purpose.

You can also catch softshells by boat. Use a small, open boat with a shallow draw (just a few inches) and pole it through the shallows, keeping a sharp lookout on the bottom for blue crabs with your net at the ready. Seining, which was described in Chapter 5, is another way to catch softshells, since you seine through shallow water.

Sometimes you can catch "future softshells" by either scapping or trapping *doublers* (a male cradle-carrying a female). As discussed in Chapter 3, when a male knows that a female is about to moult into maturity, he will carry her to the exclusion of all else (proving that humans are not the only sex-crazed creatures on earth). Occasionally doublers will conveniently stroll into a trap for you; very rarely they can also be caught by dropline. The most common way to catch doublers is by scapping them. If you do bag

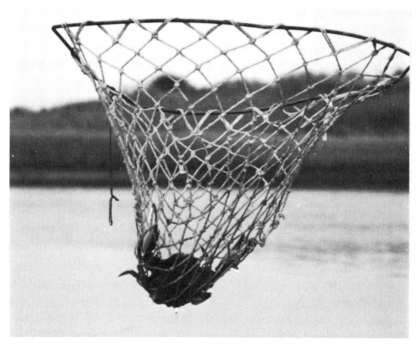

Success – a softshell from the shallows.

a doubler, separate the two soon-to-be-lovers and check the female's "signs." You could have a red sign crab on your hands. What does this mean? Read on.

When you catch blue crabs in shallow water, you can be reasonably hopeful that they're in some phase of moulting. It's up to you to determine how far along they are. Rest assured that you will also catch some big Jimmies as well, for they're going where the action is – in this case Sallies soon to be sooks and ready for mating.

It's important for you to know what moulting stage your crabs are in for several reasons. The first, and foremost, is that unknowingly mixing hardshells and softshells in a bushel basket will result in a softshell massacre. If you catch a peeler and just drop it into a bucket full of hardshells, you're not only missing a great opportunity to eat a softshell crab, you're sending that crab to certain death. If you become serious about crabbing, and enjoy softshells, use a *buster bucket.* This is simply a separate container from that which you use for the hardshells you catch. The buster bucket is for placing peelers that you catch so they can moult undisturbed. You should also have a separate bucket for true softshells as well, for the same reasons of incompatibility. If you do keep separate buckets, however, don't forget that the water in them must either be changed often or aerated to assure an adequate supply of oxygen.

It's also important to know what stage your crabs are in because papershell and buckram crabs tend to have very little meat in them. Keeping these crabs really doesn't make sense, and you would be doing yourself and other crabbers a favor by tossing them back.

Although it may sound like an impossible task to figure out what moulting stage crabs are in, it's much simpler than you think, and well worth the effort for the pleasure of dining on softshell crabs. Thanks to a blue crab's *color coding,* it's as easy to determine the moulting stage as it is to pick out a can of vegetables in the supermarket.

Before a crab begins to moult, it must first grow a soft new shell underneath its current one. You can tell when this is occurring by looking at either of the blue crab's swimming paddles. The segment above the last one on the paddles is where a thin outline of the new shell can be seen. When this outline is white in color the crab is called a *white sign,* meaning that it has approximately two weeks to go before moulting. A pink outline means the crab is a *pink sign,* and shedding will take place in about seven days. If it's red, you've got a *red sign or rank* crab, which signifies that moulting will take place in a day or so, maybe even within the next few hours.

By reading these signs you can tell how close you are to getting an honest-to-goodness softshell. Most recreational crabbers have neither the will nor the ability to shed out a white sign or even a pink sign crab, but a red sign is another story.

A crab remains a true softshell anywhere from 12 to 20 hours. Then its shell begins to harden in stages. The colorful names for these stages are: papershell, tinback or buckram, and hardshell. Each name signifies another step in the hardening process of the crab's shell.

Chapter Eight
Cooking Your Catch

Now you know how to catch hardshells and softshells. It's time to get to the payoff – the reason you went through all the trouble to catch crabs in the first place. Now it's time to talk about cooking and then eating your batch of blue crabs.

But before you can sit down to your crab feast, you've got some cooking and extracting of meat to do. (This refers to hardshell crabs; softshells need a different approach, as explained later.) While this may sound hard it's actually not, and after a few times you'll be an old hand at cooking the crab and removing its tender meat. You'll certainly be ready to try some of your own recipes; crab meat can be used in a thousand different delicious ways.

Before cooking crabs, it's always a good idea to wash them thoroughly with fresh water. Not only will this get rid of any lingering traces of seaweed or mud, it also just makes you feel better, much like washing off a piece of fruit before eating it. Crabs spend a large part of their adult lives wandering around the bottom, and unfortunately our waters are not as clean as we would like them to be. Since you can never be sure exactly where a crab's been, a little fresh water bath before cooking can't hurt.

A basement or utility room sink is a good place to wash crabs. Usually this type of sink is deep, so you can dump your crabs into it without running the risk of having them scramble out. Most kitchen sinks are shallow, and you'll be surprised how active formerly-quiet crabs will become once you dump them out of the basket. It doesn't take much for some big Jimmies to hoist themselves out of a shallow sink and begin rampaging all over the kitchen. If you don't have a basement sink, take the crabs outside and use an ordinary garden hose to clean them off.

If you didn't have your crab tongs along on the crabbing trip with you, now is the time to bring them out. With tongs you can

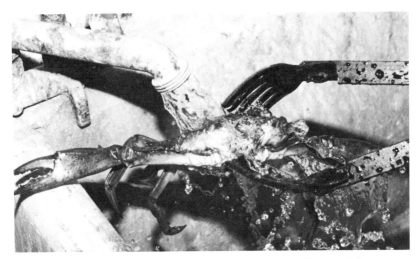

Washing off a crab before putting it into the cooking pot. Note the use of tongs once again.

easily pick up each crab individually and hold them under the water until they're cleaned to your satisfaction. Pliers, tinsnips, and similar tools are poor substitutes for tongs; not only is their gripping power inadequate, but their short handles make it easy for a cantankerous crab to draw a bead on your fingers.

After your hardshell crabs are cleaned, they're ready for the cooking pot. This is when you'll have to make the single most difficult decision in all of crabbing: to boil or to steam? Those who steam say that's the only way to go, while the boiling crowd swears by their practice. There are advantages and disadvantages to both methods.

To boil a crab, you throw it into a big pot of boiling water. Not only does this cook the crab faster, it also kills the creature instantly, and many people prefer this method because they say it's more humane.

Steaming crabs, on the other hand, requires you to put them into a pot and then slowly cook them over a moderate flame. This takes longer, both for the crab to die and for it to cook. However, steaming has one big benefit over boiling: it doesn't produce an excess amount of water in the cooked crab. When you crack open a boiled crab, there's going to be a certain amount of water that

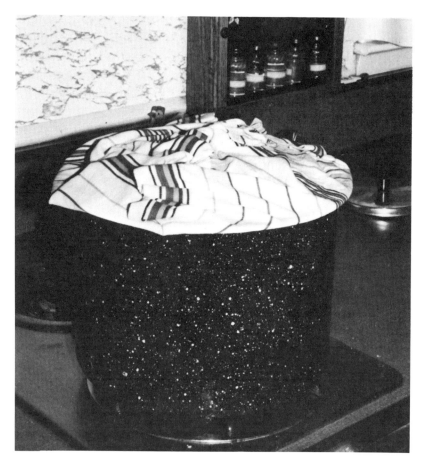

Wrapping a damp dish towel tightly around the lid of a pot is one good way to stop any steam from escaping. Be certain the towel is well away from the stove's flame.

comes flowing out, which adds to the mess that removing the meat inevitably entails. Steaming, on the other hand, eliminates this, and makes the cooked crab easier to handle.

Personally, I've always steamed my crabs. The humane argument doesn't really impact on my decision, because the crabs were caught with the intention of killing them and eating them, so the goal is the same. Everyone I know just enjoys eating crabs without having to mop up puddles of water at the same time. However, to each his own. The steam/boil controversy has been going on for a long time, and certainly isn't going to be settled in the pages of this book.

Before we get to removing the meat, a few tips: some people add a variety of spices, seasonings, etc. to the cooking pot. So do I, as you'll see by the recipe below for steamed crabs, but I've also had crabs cooked in plain old water that tasted just great. Another thing to remember is to not let cooked crabs come into contact with anything that touched the live crabs, such as the bushel basket, the tongs you used to wash them off, etc. Contamination may result.

A few people put live crabs directly into the freezer, and then cook them later. I've never tried this, primarily because it seems to leave a lot of questions unanswered about how long the crabs remain good. If you elect to try this, make sure you get all the necessary information beforehand.

No matter how you do it, eventually the crabs are going to be cooked, and then you'll have a load of bright red/orange crabs on your hands. Get your mouth ready: you're just a few minutes away from enjoying one of the truly tasty foods of all time. Just one "small" problem remains: extracting the meat from the crab. However, don't panic; it's not as difficult as it looks. In fact, if you follow the six steps listed below, you should be enjoying the savory sweet taste of blue crab in no time:

1. Pry open the apron with a sharp knife or other utensil.
2. Pull the apron around like an orange peel; this should either pop the shell off, or else loosen it so much that you can easily pull it off.
3. The whole body should now be exposed. The six sets of grayish/white, spongy material on both sides are the non-edible gills (sometimes called the devil or dead man's fingers). Remove and discard these.
4. You should be able to see some very soft material, usually yellow or green in color, just behind the mouth area. This is called the fat of the crab. Many people don't like to eat this, but some, particularly gourmets, absolutely love it. The best thing to do is to spoon it out and place it in a separate bowl, unless you're sure you don't want it, in which case you can just get rid of it.

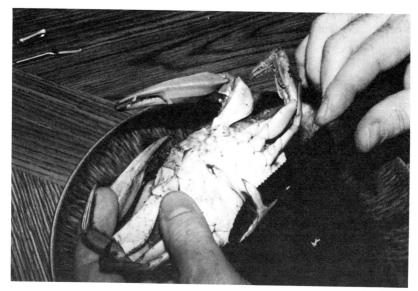

Loosening the apron.
Peeling off the shell.

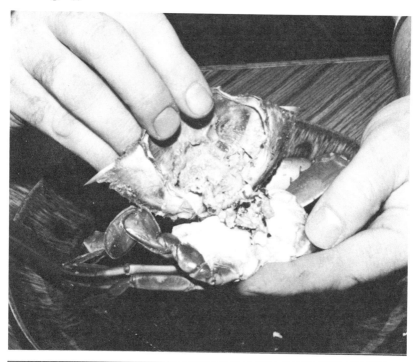

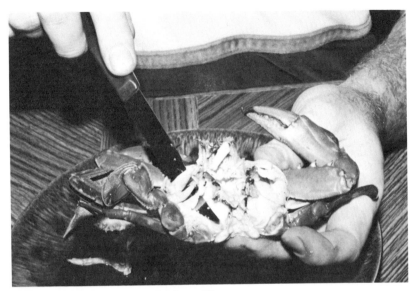

Removing the non-edible gills.

Cracking the body in half to gain better access to the meat.

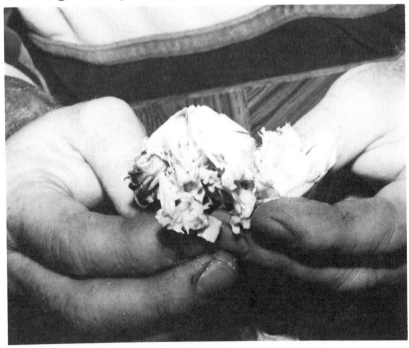

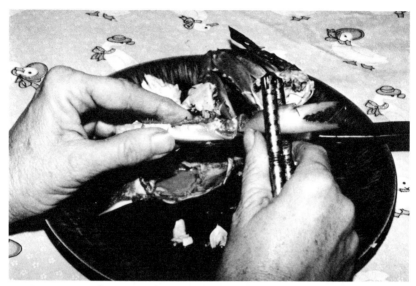

Using a cracker on the crab claws to get to the meat.

Using a nut pick to pull the meat from inside the claws.

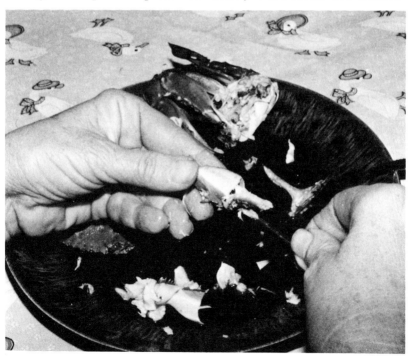

5. Next, remove the legs and claws. Some people say the claws contain the sweetest meat of all. The legs can also have a surprising amount of meat, although you'll definitely have to search for it. Use a cracker on the claws if they're too big or hurt your fingers. A nut pick or small fork can come in handy to pull out the meat from the claws and legs.

6. By now all that's left is the body of the crab. Simply break this in half. This will expose the meat underneath the white, stiff, upper membrane. You can pull this meat out using your fingers or, if you prefer to be a little more dainty (although there's nothing dainty about eating crabs) about it, with a small fork or nut pick. If you like, you can break the body sections again until the meat is easy to reach. This meat is called back-fin meat, and is it ever good!

That's all there is to it. With a little practice, you can be ripping apart your crabs with the best of them. I've seen people clean out a half-dozen big Jimmies in ten minutes or less; there's more legs flying at times like these than at a Rockettes show.

This is the classic way to eat crabs – everyone sitting around a big table laughing and talking as they crack open a pile of just-cooked crabs, the smell of the warm crabs mixing with the cooking spices and the aroma of your favorite cold beverage to create a little slice of heaven.

Use the same method to extract the meat for recipes that call for crab. However, when using crab meat for cooking, make sure to check it for stray pieces of shell or other body parts that occasionally find their way in there. No one likes suddenly crunching on a piece of shell in the midst of eating a crab cake.

Just like catching softshells was different than hardshell crabbing, cooking softshells also requires new tactics.

The first thing that's different is that you have to actually kill the softshell crab yourself before cooking, instead of letting a big pot do the dirty work. For some people this is going too far; death by cooking pot is one thing, but actually having to dispatch a crab is quite another. If you're still with me, however, there's a couple of quick methods you can use to send your softshell to Crab Heaven. The first is to jam a sharp instrument, like a knife or a small ice pick, right between the crab's eyes; the second is to chop off the entire front part of the crab, including the mouth, just behind the eyes. Of these techniques the second seems to work better, and, since you're going to have to remove the eyes and mouth before cooking anyway, why not get it all done in one fell swoop? A sharp knife or scissors does the job nicely. The area that you should be aiming for is just behind the eye stalks.

Let's assume that the softshell is now deceased. If you haven't done so already, remove the eyes and mouth. Next, loosen, but do not remove, the apron; just like with hardshells, this should also loosen the top shell, although by not taking off the apron the shell should remain connected. Now, carefully – remember, the shell is not hard – lift the shell by the two tips and clean out the gills and any other inside body material that you do not want. Then replace the shell, discard the apron, and the crab is now ready to be cooked.

Softshells are commonly fried or broiled, but, just as with hardshells, everyone has their own special recipe. Don't be afraid to experiment; crab meat is good with just about everything except breakfast cereal, and there's probably people who use it that way too. The palate you satisfy will only be your own!

Traditional Steamed Crabs
* Fill a pot with approximately one cup of water for each dozen crabs (some people mix in flat beer as well).
* Add a few capfuls of white vinegar and a generous portion of crab seasoning to the liquid.
* Place a rack or other elevated platform into the pot that clears the water on the bottom, then begin stacking crabs on top of the rack.
* After every layer, sprinkle seasoning mixture over the top of crabs; a combination of crab seasoning, salt, and spices such as Italian and/or Greek seasoning is highly recommended. When finished stacking, throw another capful or two of vinegar over everything.
* Wrap a damp dish towel around the top of the pot lid, taking care not to let any part of the towel hang down into the stove flame. The towel will keep steam from escaping, and allow your crabs to cook quicker and more completely.

* Cook crabs over a moderate flame around 20 minutes, or until they've all turned red.
* Serve with a dish of melted butter and enjoy!

Traditional Boiled Crabs
* Fill a pot about half-way with water, beer, and seasonings. Hint: throw in a touch of lemon juice for extra flavor.
* Bring water to a boil.
* Using cooking utensils, plunge each crab into the water headfirst.
* Let crabs cook about 20 minutes, or until they've turned red.
* Crack out the melted butter and get busy eating!

Traditional Fried Softshell Crabs
* One dozen cleaned softshells.
* Salt/Pepper
* Greek seasoning (if desired)
* Oil or butter

Make sure crabs are dry, then sprinkle them with salt, pepper and Greek or other desired seasoning. Fry the crabs in a skillet until brown on both sides.

Hot & Spicy Crab Cakes
* 1 lb. crab meat
* 2 tbsp. brown mustard
* 1 tbsp. Worcestershire sauce
* 1 tsp. barbecue sauce
* 1 tsp. parsley
* ¼ tsp. salt
* 1 extra large egg
* 8 tbsp. butter
* ½ cup vegetable oil

Mix the mustard, Worcestershire sauce, barbecue sauce, parsley, egg, and salt together, then add crab meat. Make the mixture into small, flat cakes, then melt the butter and oil together and fry both sides of crab cakes in it until brown. Drain and serve.

Crabmeat Cocktail
Place alternating layers of lettuce, crab meat, and cocktail sauce into a cocktail glass until full. For extra flavor try adding celery with the lettuce, or mix a few spices with crab meat.

Chapter Nine
Crab Talk

Just like any sport, crabbing has its share of unique, colorful, and (sometimes) bizarre words and phrases that sound like language from an alien civilization to those unfamiliar with the terminology. You can certainly enjoy crabbing without knowing what any of these words mean. In fact, the majority of recreational crabbers probably do not know, and could care less. However, just in case you ever encounter a leather-faced old crabber who says something like, *"Caught me a mess of doublers and buck and riders, but no shedders and only one or two peelers,"* and you'd like to be able to do more than just nod and smile at him, then the following list of crabbing terms, along with some more general words, are for you.

Colloquial Crabbing Terms . . .
Apron – the crab's abdominal region.
Buck and Rider – two crabs caught together, one on top of the other, either just before or just after mating; the buck is the male crab, the rider the female beneath him.
Buckram – the third stage of shell hardness after shedding, after papershell but before hardshell.
Buster – a crab that has just begun to "bust out" of its old shell.
Buster Bucket – a bucket into which you put hardshells that are just about to moult.
Channeler – same as a Jimmy.
Cradle Carry – when a male crab carries a female underneath him in a type of "basket" he makes with his walking legs. A cradle carry occurs either just before or just after mating.
Doubler(s) – identical to a buck and rider.
Green – same as a white sign.
Hardshell – the final stage of shell hardness.
Jimmy – a male crab.

Keeper – although its use may vary depending on what section of the country you're in, this commonly refers to a caught crab that is within the legal size limits and doesn't have to be thrown back.

Papershell – the second stage after shedding, prior to buckram but after softshell.

Peeler – usually means when a crab is just about ready to shed its old shell.

Pink Sign – a crab that has about one week to go before moulting.

Rank – a crab that is ready to shed its shell (moult).

Red Sign – same as rank.

Sally – an immature female crab (one that is not yet capable of producing eggs).

Scapping – catching crabs without bait, by just using a long-handled scoop/dip net.

She-Crab – same as a sook.

Shedder – a crab that is actively engaged in coming out of its old shell.

Snot – same as a white sign.

Softshell – when a crab has totally shed its old shell and now has a soft shell.

Sook – a mature female crab.

Sponge Crab – a female crab that is carrying a highly visible mass of eggs on her abdomen in a sac that looks like a large sponge.

Tinback – same as a buckram.

White – same as a white sign.

White Sign – a crab that has about two weeks to go before moulting.

Words For the Scientists Among You . . .

Breaking planes – the points along a crab's appendages at which breakage can occur without injury to the crab.

Callinectes sapidus – the "proper" name for the blue crab; can be loosely translated as "beautiful savory swimmer."

Carapace – a crab's shell.

Chela – a crab's claw.

Chitin – what a crab's shell and external body is made of.

Crustaceans – the classification into which crabs belong, which means animals whose soft bodies are covered by a hard outer covering, and who have jointed appendages and gills.

Megalops – the larval stage of a crab before it metamorphoses into what we recognize as a crab; the word means "large eyes."

Moulting – the scientific term for a crab shedding its shell.

Regeneration – the process by which a crab can grow a new appendage to take the place of one that was lost.

Zoea – the microscopic larval stage of a crab immediately after hatching.

Chapter Ten
A Crabbing Tale

The first pink rays of sunlight were just peeking over the horizon when we clambered into the car, trying desperately not to make any noise at that early morning hour but of course making some anyway, as we slammed car doors and banged our nets and crab traps into the trunk. On our drive to the dock, my father, grandfather, and I witnessed a world just waking up: sleepy-eyed paper boys tossing morning papers onto lawns (or into rose bushes), a few "early birds" streaking across the slowly-brightening sky, and street lights winking out in response to the coming day. Although it was mid-July, the heat and humidity of the day were still asleep; the air was cool, moist, and refreshing. It was a perfect day for crabbing.

Down at the water's edge, the docks were swarming with activity, as they usually were early in the morning. Fishermen were firing up their ship's engines, people were queuing up to the bait counter in steady streams, and teenage boys were hurrying from one small rowboat to another, gassing up the tiny outboards and making sure there were enough flotation cushions in each boat. The contrast between everyday life and the docks was always fascinating; it was like two different worlds – one still asleep, the other energetically awake – separated by nothing but a few feet of road.

But even as I filled my lungs with the good, clean salt air, my mind drifted to the significance of today's crabbing trip. It was going to be the first time I had ever worked droplines by myself from a boat – a tall order for an eight-year-old boy.

While my father took care of the business of renting us a boat (since he always was the one who had to row it all over the river, he might as well get one he liked), my grandfather and I unloaded the lines, sinkers, traps, and nets from the car. At this stage of his life my grandfather was a large, stocky man, with a thick thatch of white hair and a smile that crinkled up the corners of his eyes. He looked at me and smiled; I smiled back, somewhat nervously. Once we were out on the water, there was little discussion about where to go. My grandfather always had everything worked out days beforehand. Like an ancient alchemist he would consult tide schedules, nautical charts, and phases of the moon diagrams, until he found the exact time and place that would yield the most crabs. I never knew him to be wrong.

Crabbing to him was like a religion. Certain parts of it were sacrosanct, such as never taking either a mature female or a crab that was below his self-imposed limit of five inches tip-to-tip (although the law was more lenient). He also didn't believe in using crab traps, or anything else besides a dropline. To him a dropline represented the ultimate contest: man against crab – no strings attached. He brought traps along for my dad and I, but would deliberately avoid pulling them up, as if to even touch a single one would brand him for life as a "trapper."

At droplining my grandfather was a master. He'd always know when there was a crab on his line, even though the bait sat submerged and unseen in the brackish water and the current was constantly jerking the line to and fro. All my grandfather would have to do is gently grasp his line between his thumb and forefinger, like a doctor feeling for a pulse. Then he would either nod or else slip the line back into the water.

When he nodded that he had a "customer," the real contest would begin. By using just two fingers he could wind the line around his hand, bringing it up in one smooth, continuous motion, without causing a single ripple in the glass-like surface of the water. He took his time doing this, with a slight smile creasing his well-worn face and all his attention focused on the string slowly rising out of the water like some aquatic elevator heading for the penthouse. In his other hand he lightly held his ancient wooden-handled scoop net that always seemed as big as a telephone pole to me.

Just when I was certain that he'd pulled the bait up too far, and that the crab was long gone, his net would swoop down. When the net came back up it would inevitably have a blue crab in it; it always gave me a feeling of immense pleasure to see the crab's olive-green shell glistening in the summer sun.

From the time of my very first crabbing trip, my grandfather tried to teach me his dropline technique. Since being a kid means having too little patience and too much energy, I would quickly tire of the tedious, almost somnambulistic pace of handlining and go back to my traps, where all it took was one quick yank to achieve the same result.

Little by little, however, I fell under the dropline's spell. Each time the three of us went out I would spend more and more time working on bringing up the line slowly and smoothly. If you do it long enough, it gets in your blood.

On that day when I was to handle my own droplines, my father rowed us to the spot pinpointed by my grandfather – a quiet, out of the way backwater channel where our only company was the squawking of gulls perched on some rotted pilings nearby, the remnants of a long-gone dock. Then both he and my grandfather busied themselves with their own lines. Clearly I was on my own.

I painstakingly baited two lines, put a small sinker on each, and dropped them over the side. It was early in the morning, about six o'clock; the sun was still low on the eastern horizon. A cool breeze skipped over the water. It was the ideal time for catching crabs.

My grandfather hit first, as he always seemed to do. He pulled in what he called a "double-header" on his line – two crabs going after the same bait. The big male was unceremoniously dumped into our bushel basket; the female, large and, by a quick look at her apron, sexually mature, was tossed back, accompanied by my grandfather's usual comment: "Go back and make us some more crabs, Missy."

Maybe it was because he was originally from the city that my grandfather loved and respected the water so much. Long before the word "environmental" came into vogue my grandfather policed the water in his own fashion, using his scoop net to hoist floating debris out and insisting that we always use a rowboat, not a motor boat, because of the pollutants discharged by even the tiniest outboard engines.

His biggest crusade, however, concerned throwing back "baby" crabs. He would get positively apoplectic at people who routinely kept small crabs, some measuring little more than two inches. To him that was suicide, not only for the crab population but for the sport of crabbing too.

That day, there was a lot of throwing back little ones. Both my father and grandfather seemed to be giving back as many as they took. But at least they were pulling something in, unlike me. Several times I had felt my lines, hefting each string in my fingers to see if there were any unusual vibrations coming from either one. Each time the lines were silent. Enviously I watched my father and grandfather pull in crabs as if using a vacuum. It's always hard to be a wallflower, especially at a three-man party.

Just when I was giving serious thought to chucking the whole thing and going back to my traps, my grandfather, staring out at the open water, said quietly: "Crabs don't always announce themselves, you know."

I knew exactly what he meant. Sometimes crabs will hit on your bait with nary a vibration at all, just sit there on the bottom and daintily pick it apart while you wonder why you haven't gotten even a nibble. My grandfather was telling me to pull my lines up even if I didn't think anything was on them.

The instant I pulled the bait off the bottom from my first line I felt the familiar jerking tugs that signal a crab is coming along for the ride. For the first time in my life, I felt that curious quickening of the heart that always occurs when a blue crab strikes. It's a type of apprehensive excitement, fueled by the myriad of uncertainties that race through every crabber's mind as they bring up their bait: How big is the crab? Will it drop off just as I'm about to net it? What if it's a big one and I miss it?

In the time it took for those questions to go racing through my mind I had lifted half the line out of the water. I thought I could make out a vague white shape a few feet down in the water; that would be the bait. But what was that floating object right next to it?

To me it looked like the world's biggest crab.

Not daring to take my eyes off it, I grabbed blindly for my scoop net and knocked it to the floor of the boat, where it hit with a sound like two trains colliding. Since crabs are not fond of loud noises, I was certain that the crash would send my giant jetting away. But, incredibly, it was still there, swimming next to my bait and tearing hunks off with its claws.

Of course, without my scoop net it was going to be difficult to land the crab. Suddenly there was a slight pressure on my left leg; someone had put another scoop net there. I shot a quick look at my father and grandfather, but they were both staring intently down at their lines as if they had a gold bar on the other end. Carefully this time, I picked up my net, then slid it into the water. The crab and bait were about a foot and one-half away from the surface – the critical point at which you either net the crab or it takes off. Even though the water distorts everything, making small crabs seem big, this one *was* big. Of that I was certain.

I held my breath and scooped. My eyes might have even been closed.

"I got him, I got him!" I cried as I lifted the net out of the water. And indeed I had; lying flat in the net, its claws folded close to its body, was a good-sized blue crab. Not the record-breaking giant I had imagined, but certainly large enough to be labeled a "big one" by everyone in our family.

Now my father and grandfather sprang into action, helping me bring the net over the boat before I dropped it, crab and all, into the water in my delirium. For about five seconds I was on top of the world, as they congratulated me and I imagined the hero's welcome that I would receive from my hungry aunts, uncles and cousins who always gathered at our home whenever they knew we were going crabbing. Then, in unison, my father and grandfather said: "Uh oh."

My eyes flew to my captive crab. Still in the net, it had flipped over on its back in its struggle to get free, revealing a thick, brownish, gelatin-like mass bulging from its underside.

"Sponge crab," my grandfather said simply.

I immediately knew that my first solo catch on a dropline would have to go back. We would all rather jump naked into a bucket of angry crabs than take a female ready to give birth.

But I didn't feel too badly as I watched the expectant mother slip beneath the surface of the water and back to her freedom. I had, after all, caught her by myself, despite her "delicate condition." More importantly, I had proven that, while not by any means a master of the dropline, I was at least a competent pupil.

Thus would the circle remain unbroken – a tradition that had begun with my grandfather's father would be continued down through me.

It's been many a year now since my grandfather and I shared a rowboat together, but I think about that tradition often as I watch my young daughter trying to master the skills of droplining, as the sun sparkles off the water and the squawking of gulls echoes in the misty distance. A tradition is so much better if you have someone to share it with.

Other Books by Centennial Publications

Colorado Classic Cane
A History of the Colorado Bamboo Rod Makers
By Dick Spurr & Michael Sinclair

In Over My Waders
Flyfishing Humor
By Gray Ugly

Dickerson: The Man and His Rods
By Gerald S. Stein and James W. Schaaf

Classic Bamboo Rodmakers – Past and Present
By Dick Spurr

The Bamboo Rod And How to Build It
By Claude M. Kreider

Making and Using The Dry Fly
With Valuable Notes On Leaders and Stream Tactics
By Paul H. Young

Wes Jordan: Profile of a Rodmaker
Cross – South Bend – Orvis
By Dick Spurr & Gloria Jordan

Montague Rod & Reel Co. Reproduction Catalog

The E. F. Payne Rod Co. Corporate Record Book
1930 – 1968